Is food an overwhelming part of your life?

FOOD FOR LOVE:
Healing the Food, Sex, Love
& Intimacy Relationship

This groundbreaking new recovery guide helps us peel back years of overeating, diets, and binges to uncover the causes of our eating problems. Through her own life story and those of her patients, psychologist Janet Greeson shows how unresolved losses—such as a loss of trust in someone important, physical or emotional abuse as a child, negative childhod messages about sex, an emotionally distant parent—can sap our spirit and cut us off from our fullest selves. Janet Greeson's powerful ninety-day program opens the path to discovering:

- how we may be using food to express unspoken feelings.
- how repressed secrets lead to compulsive overeating—and how to escape from the vicious cycle.
- how trust, identity, and self-image can be shattered in childhood or later in life—and how to begin the healing process.
- how to regain the comfort of self-trust—and meet intimacy needs from a platform of self-respect.
- how to liberate the spirit within—and respond fully and joyfully to life.

As food takes its proper place in our lives, we can begin to enjoy it in a healthful new way—and experience the richest satisfactions of a truly abundant life.

Also by Janet Greeson

It's Not What You're Eating, It's What's Eating You
Food for Love

FOOD FOR LOVE
HEALING THE FOOD, SEX, LOVE & INTIMACY RELATIONSHIP

JANET GREESON, Ph.D.

POCKET BOOKS

New York   London   Toronto   Sydney   Tokyo   Singapore

POCKET BOOKS, a division of Simon & Schuster Inc.
1230 Avenue of the Americas, New York, NY 10020

Copyright © 1993 by Janet Greeson and Catherine Revland

ISBN: 0-671-78310-6

First Pocket Books printing March 1994

10 9 8 7 6 5 4 3 2 1

POCKET and colophon are registered trademarks of Simon & Schuster Inc.

Printed in the U.S.A.

"Simple Gifts," adapted by Aaron Copland, Boosey & Hawkes, Inc., Publisher

Contents

Contents

vii

Preface

There are a thousand different programs for losing weight that are logical and should work, but they don't. Eventually they all fail because they address only a small part of the problem—how we look—while ignoring the real problem—how we feel. How we feel is not just about a discontentment with our bodies, but a chronic state of detachment from life, a sense of disconnection from others, and most of all, a disconnection from ourselves. Obviously, a weight loss program that does not treat such deep and unhappy feelings is destined to fail, especially when those feelings are often what drive us to food in the first place.

Patients often come into treatment unable to describe this disconnected state they are in. Ask them how they feel, and they will tell you, "I don't know." At first it is difficult for them to grasp the meaning of disconnection because the part that is missing cannot be seen, heard, or felt, only experienced. It is a part of themselves they may not even know exists. It is their spirit.

This spirit is the source of our internal energy. People who have a lot of it are expansive, magnetic, joyful, inspiring, even larger than life. Actual size has nothing to do with the amount of energy a person has. George Burns and Michael Jackson are enormous in spirit. In fact, it is when we are at our smallest that our energy is the most intense. If you have ever watched a row of newborns in any hospital nursery, you will understand what I mean.

Disconnected people have lost their spirit, that incredible energy that emanates from us and that we are all born with. Its loss is what depression and boredom are really about. If you are in the presence of disconnected people, you will experience their loss—they leave you feeling exhausted and you don't know why.

Disconnected people can no longer respond to the normal sensory stimulations of life. It's as if their bodies can receive messages, but their sense organs can't send them on to be experienced. Disconnected people can't be stirred by a particular color or the shape of a cloud, the sound of the rain or a saxophone riff, or the fragrance of a rose. They can't feel exhilarated in the exchange of energy that comes from being connected to others in a meaningful way.

Disconnected people are unable to feel even when good things happen to them. If they win a prize or an award, they go through the motions of being excited, but inside they feel next to nothing. When unhappy things happen, they feel the same numbness. They are detached from their surroundings and become onlookers in their own lives, repressing the deep feelings of sadness, loss, anger, loneliness, and grief that should be expressed.

In an attempt to escape from the boredom of their flattened emotional landscape, disconnected people become sensation seekers. Because they are numb, they look for intensity; it is the only way they can feel anything. Sensation seekers go for the thrill. They want to be shocked rather than stimulated. They need to be oversensitized: A funny joke becomes hysterical; fondness turns into passion; a sad story evokes a torrent of weeping. Just as the hearing impaired need to turn up the volume in order to hear at all, so the feeling impaired need to turn up the intensity in order to feel at all.

Many disconnected people talk about how they experienced heightened emotion for the first time with the help of alcohol, a drug, other people, work, gambling, food—whatever form an addiction takes. Invariably they describe that first euphoric moment as if it were an epiphany: "So this is what it means to be alive!" Before the event, life was flat and gray and meant nothing. Afterward, as long as the outside source of energy was available, life was exciting and everything was possible. No wonder addictions are so important to disconnected people!

The mind's ability to numb the body and prevent it from being able to feel a heightened experience is a serious kind of sensory starvation. It is the perpetually unresolved quest for the full experience that propels the addiction, and it is why no amount is ever enough.

Food as an addictive choice has many things in its favor: It is safe, readily available, and socially acceptable, especially at the family dinner table, where food and love are forever merged. No wonder there are so many people these days who find themselves addicted to food. I could make a good case for calling it the primal addiction. Over and over again I have heard people tell how an addiction to food came roaring forth after they gave up their alcohol and drugs, their cigarettes, workaholism, or unhealthy relationships.

Food is particularly well suited to fill the addictive craving for intensity as it is connected to the infantile experience when all sensations were heightened. Food is also emotionally charged. As children, food and love were taken in blindly from the same source. It's inevitable that strong feeling attached to food would have to be experienced by addicts in a distorted way. For us, food carries an emotional weight far heavier than anything that can be measured in calories or grams. There was a time when eating was too important in my life. I distorted a deep need for comfort and understanding into the way I felt about certain foods. Just the sight of a plate of mashed potatoes could move me to tears if I was feeling bad, and I always felt cozy and warm as I ate it, as if a friendly arm was around my shoulder.

The ways food addicts distort their relationship with food run the gamut of emotional needs, from comfort to lust. For many, the distortion is romantic. They describe the relationship using the words and gestures of a lover. Food evokes not just pleasure in the way it tastes and smells, but elicits passion, excitement, even danger, as the relationship frequently takes the form of a love affair. What or how much is consumed becomes a well-kept secret. There is a further distortion around the peak sensations, which tend to occur not while eating the food, but in the anticipation phase. Sometimes the intensity of this phase becomes so unbearable food addicts will tear into the grocery bags and start eating on the way home from the store.

I have noticed that a passionate feeling about food is especially prevalent among adults who are sexually shut down because of childhood abuse. All those intense feelings have to go somewhere, and food is a particularly safe outlet because another person does not have to be involved.

For a while, food does carry the heavy emotional burdens we give it, although not without the consequences of extra weight. Like all addictions, however, overstimulation will ultimately bring about the opposite of the desired effect in the form of a sensory shutdown. The body becomes more and more desensitized until one day the thrill is gone and the addictive substance no longer works. Like a battery that has died, the substance or activity no longer provides the energy charge needed, and this deprivation leaves the disconnected person even more helpless and numb. A patient once described that feeling as "falling through emptiness." It motivates a lot of people to seek help for a situation that can no longer be tolerated, and they will even take desperate measures to change.

How This Book Can Help

Food for Love: Healing the Food, Sex, Love, & Intimacy Relationship is for people who feel they are disconnected, who have become numb to the enjoyment of life and other people and have turned to food to experience the heightened emotion they crave. The program in this book involves no desperate measures, but it does involve change, small and daily, for ninety days. We may need to lose weight, but first we must retrieve our lost and hungry spirit.

Ten percent of our being is in the realm of the physical, the body and all its cravings, the part where an addiction lies. It is the part of ourselves that we show to the world at large, but it is only a small part of who we really are. Thirty percent of our being is in the realm of the mind—our thoughts, feelings, and intellect. It is our cognitive self, the part that can reason, rationalize, and process all the information we receive daily. However, it can also confuse, distort, or deny this information. It is the part of us that knows six good reasons why the piece of fruit on the dessert cart is the right choice but still reaches for the cake. It is the part that can twist reality when the truth is too threatening. It can even trick the body in order to protect itself. It is this 30 percent that makes us believe that the addictive substance can satisfy our needs, the part that convinces our body that it is the best way to experience pleasure.

The 60 percent that remains is our spirit, that remarkable energy source that is our essence and brings wonder and joy to everything we do. Unlike our cognitive self that can distort reality or our body that can be tricked with artificial stimulus, the spirit cannot exist in an environment it perceives as unsafe. Instead, when it is attacked or threatened, the spirit retreats and buries itself deep inside. We repress our spirit as a means of self-defense—we don't want to feel hurt or vulnerable—but we wind up feeling nothing at all. We live an incomplete life—we're living with only forty percent of our being!

The goal of my first book, *It's Not What You're Eating, It's What's Eating You,* was to free a person from the prison of addiction. With its twenty-eight-day food and activity plan, the emphasis was on the needs of the body and mind, the former to become cleansed and detoxified and the latter to respond to a modification of behavior and a reorienting of thinking. In *Food for Love,* it is the needs of the spirit that take priority: We must nourish and protect it so it can thrive again and become powerful.

If your spirit has been in hiding a long time, it needs a slow and steady readjustment to the light of day. Every day for ninety days, you will be taking an action that nourishes your spirit, feeds it good thoughts, and tends to its needs and desires in a loving way. By focusing on the needs of the spirit, I think you will be amazed at how the needs of the mind and body take care of themselves.

If you have a problem with an addiction of any kind, you can still use this ninety-day program. I strongly recommend that beginning with Day One you remove all addictive substances from your diet, including caffeine, white flour, and refined sugars of all kinds, as they trigger the addictive impulse of always wanting more, and they have been linked to depression and mood swings.

The program is constructed around the ninety-meetings-in-ninety-days recovery model, with or without twelve-step meetings. Although group meetings such as Overeaters Anonymous or other twelve-step meetings are not necessary to use this program, I highly recommend them to accelerate recovery. If you have read my first book, you will find this program will take you further on in your journey.

I would like you to think of the next ninety days as a time when your spirit is in intensive care. When it has been restored, you can go out and have a wonderful life with meaning, purpose, and excitement, but right now you have some nurturing to do. If you should miss a day, don't fret. Rigidity is part of the problem. However, don't use a lapse as an excuse to fail; resume your activities the next day.

These daily activities are action oriented. They will help you change the way you feel about yourself. In the process, they will change the way other people experience you. The activities can be done alone, but many involve the real world and changing your interactions with significant people in your life today. The actions you will be taking will improve and deepen these relationships. Other activities will help you access memories and the secret messages they contain that are at the core of what's eating you.

The first step of recovery involves discovery of the source of disconnection and retrieval of the deeply buried unexpressed feelings around this source. More than the actual event, however, it's these unexpressed feelings that have been repressed that are the real problem. We expend all our energy burying these emotions and in the process shut down our capacity to feel anything at all.

The next step is expressing those buried feelings. Tears cried alone are not enough. The feelings must be acknowledged by others in order for them to be released and their powerful negative energy diffused. You need to find someone you can trust and who understands you in order to achieve maximum benefit from this book—a therapist, husband, mother or father, brother or sister, friend or support group member—someone you feel close to who has good energy and truly cares about you.

If your depression has isolated you to the point where there is no one you can trust, don't give up. Begin the journey knowing that your need will be met. If you seek someone to believe in you, that person will appear in your life.

The goal of reconnection is a treasure beyond

value. It is the emergence of the person you really are, a person who is not afraid to feel and radiates an energy other people find exciting. It will be a gradual reconnection. One day you will look around you and realize that your life has become exciting because once again you are open to experiencing its many small pleasures in a complete way. You will experience heightened sensations as they were created to be experienced: in mind and body, without denial or distortion, permeating your entire being, touching the Real You—your spirit.

When you have achieved the goal of reconnection, you will see life with a new clarity and purpose. Suddenly you know who you are and your energy is around that identity, not scattered in every direction as it was before. You will know you are someone to be loved and valued, not for anything said or done, but just for being. This true self is the great treasure that lies buried within us, which awaits our discovery so that we may have a rich and meaningful life.

The reconnection you seek may come within the ninety days of this program or on the journey that follows. It doesn't matter when it comes, only that it does come, for it is what will bring you the energy that makes life meaningful and magical. The process of recovery cannot be speeded up, but neither can it be stopped. If you keep putting one foot ahead of the other and keep your spirit's urgent needs close to your heart while you do the program's daily activities, I'm promising you it will work for you in ways you have yet to dream of.

FOOD FOR LOVE

I

Food for Love

Jenny grew up an only child in a comfortable home where a voice raised in anger was rare. Her parents were loving and kind. She had an idyllic childhood as the youngest of six cousins who spent their summers at her grandparents' farm in rural Alabama. The early 1960s was a time of civil strife turmoil, and in nearby Montgomery little girls like herself were being bombed in churches, but Jenny's world was safe and wonderful. Her earliest memory is being passed adoringly among the laps of aunts, uncles, and cousins, a long-awaited, longed-for child. Jenny describes the most exciting moment of her life as being eight years old, swinging over a pond on a tire swing her grandfather had strung over a high branch of a giant oak tree and finally getting up the courage to let go. She can still hear the cheers and the applause of her cousins as she soared through the air and splashed into the water.

1

FOOD FOR LOVE

Jenny's parents were very modern and educated. They were health care advocates, active in their community of Fort Green, Brooklyn. They went through Lamaze training for her birth and were careful never to inhibit their little daughter because she was a girl. (In fact, Jenny grew up to be an electrical engineer.) They were very much opposed to corporal punishment of children and did not even like the idea of raising one's voice harshly. Instead, when Jenny misbehaved, they withdrew their affection and ignored her, as if she were invisible.

The summer Jenny was eleven, her mother and father came into her room one evening at bedtime. She can still vividly recall the pineapple carving on her canopy bedpost and the pink tufted bedspread her parents sat on. Quietly, gently, and without emotion, they told her that daddy and mommy had decided not to live together anymore. From now on, Jenny would live with her mother during the week and see her father on the weekends in his new apartment in the city. It had, they said, a wonderful view.

In that quiet moment on her bed, Jenny's world shattered. Aside from the shock of meeting her father's girlfriend, she remembers little of the events that followed. Jenny had been told (or she chose to hear) that the separation was "only for a while," and she began praying and making wishes every night that her parents would get back together. Because her mother and father had always acted so pleasantly toward each other when they were around her, Jenny had truly believed her fervent prayers and magic spells were working. However, it wasn't long before her father married his girlfriend, destroying any hopes that Jenny had of her parents reconciling.

Of course, Jenny never voiced her feelings of rage, betrayal, and loss over her perfect childhood, her anger at feeling as if her whole world had been pulled out from under her without warning. In her family, it was unthinkable to express any strong feelings. When Jenny recalls that time of her life, she sees herself at a window looking up and down the street for her daddy or sitting by the telephone waiting for it to ring. She felt abandoned and alone and withdrew into herself.

Jenny never told anyone how much hurt and anger she was feeling. Instead, she began to steal from her new stepmother. She took change and dollar bills from her purse and wore her diamond earrings to school on several occasions. One day her stepmother's good jewelry box was gone from her dresser drawer and she stopped leaving money in her purse, but no one ever said a word to Jenny about what was going on. Everyone acted as if nothing had ever happened.

The following year, thirteen-year-old Jenny and her mother moved to California. She missed her family and friends and felt like a stranger when she visited her father's house. He and his new wife were beginning a family of their own, and her father gave her less and less attention. Jenny shut down. She made fewer and fewer demands on her father's time in order to protect herself from disappointment and the agony of waiting for him. She was lonely. She didn't know how to connect with people at her new school or in the neighborhood. Jenny excused her failure to make friends by telling herself that as an only child and the youngest of her extended family, she had never learned how to connect with others her own age. She had always felt "not old enough."

For years Jenny went through the motions of having a life. She studied hard and excelled at school, had many acquaintances but no real friends—no one she was intimate with. Jenny felt she didn't fit in. Californians had beautiful bodies and were good at outdoor sports, whereas she was hopelessly unathletic and liked to be indoors. She excelled in and even enjoyed what nearly everyone else her age hated and shunned—math. The "cool" kids didn't pay any attention to her, and Jenny wanted nothing to do with the "nerds," who like herself were interested only in math and science. So she spent most of her time with her mother. During the week, mother and daughter would spend their nights in front of the television, and on weekends the two of them would get into the car and just drive around. Her mother would laugh grimly about their aimless excursions and say, "Well, it's hard to get lost if you don't have a destination." During these trips Jenny's mother would make other jokes about being the cast-off wife and finished with life. She would also tell Jenny "the facts of life"— how all men were untrustworthy and would eventually abandon her. The more time she spent with her mother, the more Jenny identified with her, and soon she, too, felt old and used up.

Jenny's separation from her father and extended family and the sudden disruption of her perfect life were the sources of her depression; her mother's negative messages reaffirmed and intensified her feelings of abandonment. Jenny isolated herself more and more and began to shut out the world around her. Her life became empty and numb, a mechanical process without emotions.

Then, at age twenty-five, with a Ph.D. and a new job, Jenny fell madly in love. Instead of having no feelings, they went out of control. However, even in the early euphoric stages of her love affair, a little voice told her it would not last. Her lover was an executive in another department and a married man with small children. He also traveled on business a great deal. Jenny saw him so infrequently that she realized one day with a sickening feeling in the pit of her stomach that she had fallen back into her old pattern that had begun with her parents' separation, of waiting for a telephone that didn't ring. At that moment Jenny knew that she had fallen in love with a man who was as emotionally unavailable as her father, right down to his preoccupation with young children.

Jenny had no one to turn to for comfort. For once she truly regretted having no close friends. She couldn't talk to either parent about how she felt. Her mother would only use her unhappy experience as an excuse for another lecture about the shortcomings of men and the terrible status of women in this society. Although Jenny loved her mother very much and they were deeply bonded, she always came away from contact with her feeling tainted, wearing her mother's feelings of low value and undesirability and tasting her mother's bitterness on her tongue. As for her father, Jenny hadn't felt intimate with him for years. When they were together, they treated each other with superficial cheer. She could never spoil their precious time together by telling him her troubles. She wanted him to think she was really happy, because he had always told her that was the only thing he had ever wanted for her.

Jenny had to look elsewhere for something to make her feel better. More and more she turned to food. It had to be a certain kind of food, though. Jenny's special food was pudding. She would even get in her car and drive miles in the middle of the night to a twenty-four-hour supermarket to buy some if she was suffering from a particularly bad bout of emptiness.

When she and her mother had first moved to California and money was short, they used to buy boxes of pudding mix on sale. In the evenings, Jenny or her mother would open a package of pudding mix, pour it into a saucepan, add the milk, and then cook it on the stove, stirring it with a wooden spoon until it thickened.

"Making the pudding" became a ritual of increasing importance in their life. It became an every-night snack they spooned down together while watching their favorite show, reruns of "The Odd Couple." They made a game of it: Monday was chocolate; Tuesday was vanilla; and Wednesday, butterscotch. Sometimes Jenny would take two different flavors cooked up in separate batches and marbleize them together in a bowl, swirling with her spoon to blend the flavors.

Eating the pudding also became a ritual. Mother and daughter would sit side by side on the living room couch that had come with them from their old apartment and laugh quietly at the mishaps of Oscar and Felix. A few commercials into the show, Jenny would start to feel warm and cozy, the way she felt as a little child when, in her pajamas and ready for bed, she would sit for a while between her parents on the living room couch and watch TV. To feel warm and cozy again, if only for a few minutes, was what pudding was all about. Understand the greatness of Jenny's loss: Her childish naiveté, her protected view of life as a place where nothing could go wrong, had been ripped away like a blanket on a cold night, and a part of her was still shivering. It took pudding to get her through the time when she felt the coldest— the time when she needed to be warm and have her memories glow the brightest. When she swallowed it slowly, spoonful by silken, quivery spoonful, she felt safe and protected. She didn't know why she got comfort from that particular taste and texture; all she knew was that when the bad feelings in her head wouldn't go away, her body screamed, "Pudding!"

In college Jenny had discovered ready-made pudding snacks in two- and four-serving packs in the supermarket dairy case. She loved those pudding snacks. She loved the way the foil curled back when she peeled off the sealed top of each little plastic portion, and she was nearly overcome when one day she discovered the two-tone packages of pudding—chocolate on the bottom and vanilla on top—that she could swirl together like in her high school days, snacking with her mother. Most of all, she loved the fact that the pudding was ready to eat—instant gratification. Some nights when she was feeling really low, she would be ashamed to see how many of those white plastic cups were in the garbage. One day as she ripped the cardboard off a new pack, she laughed ironically at the phrase "Serves four." She never shared her pudding anymore. Unfortunately, eating just one of those portions and saving the rest for later was an impossibility. More and more, it took the whole box to produce the warm and cozy feelings she craved. One day she stepped onto the scale at her doctor's office and was shocked to find she had gained forty pounds, most of it pudding.

Jenny's breakup with her married boyfriend was both painful and prolonged, but she had to leave him because she couldn't tolerate the infrequency of their times together or the way holidays made her feel because he had to be with his family. Most of all, she couldn't stand waiting for the phone to ring. Her lover had no reason to want to change the status quo and kept trying to persuade her to resume the relationship until Jenny finally had to change her number to an unlisted one. Her loneliness was greater than ever before, and by now the pudding could hardly make a dent in it.

Jenny's state of disconnection was like a bottom-less chasm, a condition so profound and yet so ordinary she barely acknowledged it. She would often think about her extended family and how much she missed them. Except for funerals, she rarely saw her grandparents, aunts, uncles, and cousins anymore. They always remarked that it was a pity that the only time they got together anymore was for such a sad occasion. However, year after year they did nothing to get the family together, mainly for reasons of geography but also for lack of real connection in their everyday lives.

Jenny yearned for the old days. At holiday time, if she ran across a photo in a magazine of people smiling around a festive dining room table, she would sometimes surprise herself by bursting into tears. The scattering of her extended family was no one's fault, but somehow the loss felt like a betrayal.

What Jenny missed the most was also the least attainable—the times when she and her relatives did nothing special together, maybe just sit on the back porch listening to the crickets or clean out the garage. It was that daily ordinariness of her connections with family that she yearned for the deepest.

Six months after Jenny's breakup with the married man, a new engineering department was opened up. In the scramble of personnel, she found herself sharing an office with a handsome and charming man who found her very attractive. Unfortunately, he was also married. At least this time, she told herself, he had no children. Although her new man insisted he liked his women on the heavy side, Jenny immediately went on a liquid diet and lost 20 pounds. Their affair was short-lived and ultimately humiliating. His wife had nearly caught them in bed together. Three months into the relationship, her lover was sent to Asia, and Jenny felt rescued and devastated at the same time.

A stray dog wandered into her life, and she nurtured it back to health. She withdrew completely and felt she had nothing to look forward to except work, eating, and the dog she named Fidelity because "She's true to me no matter what."

Unable to find a source for the comfort she needed in her relationships, Jenny turned with increasing desperation to food. To her despair, however, she found that the greater her need, the less food satisfied her emotional cravings. After she had spooned down that first smooth and creamy portion of pudding, all the following portions did was make her feel full, then foolish, and, finally, angry at herself for having no self-control, eating and eating even though she was no longer hungry, and sabotaging yet another battle to try to control her food intake.

For years Jenny had been waging this war against her appetite, especially the late-night "snack attacks" on her vigilance. What did it matter how much she stuck to her diet during the day when every night, between nine and bedtime, she went wild in the kitchen? Little by little, she gave up dieting altogether.

As the months went by and Jenny became heavier and lonelier and more reliant on food to comfort herself, she reached a point where it felt as if food took over. It wasn't so much what she consumed but that she felt she was being consumed—by her obsession with food. Eating had become life instead of being a part of living. Most disturbing of all was how food no longer filled her emotional needs. No amount of pudding could get her into that warm and cozy place she yearned for.

With the loss of her last available source of comfort, Jenny went into a panic and sought help. "What's wrong with me?" she would berate herself. "I've always had a good life—easy compared to most people. My parents got divorced, but so did most everyone's parents when I was growing up. I have a great mom and dad and even a nice stepmother. I've been blessed with brains and talent, I have my degree and a good job and money in the bank. Why am I so unhappy? And why is the only thing I could always depend on to feel better—food—now my worst enemy? How can I get out of this miserable rut I'm in?"

You Can't Get Enough of What You Don't Need

Like Jenny, I used to turn to food to fill my deepest emotional needs. I too craved something soft and smooth. The source of my good feelings was mashed potatoes. One of my most intensely pleasurable early memories of food is watching my dad sit at the kitchen table and make mashed potatoes on his plate. Whenever my mother served them boiled whole or cut in halves, my father would mash the boiled potatoes with his fork, add a chunk of butter and a little milk, and stir it around until it was smooth and creamy. I would do the same to my potatoes and always held each forkful in my mouth for a while before swallowing it.

I believe I have this very pleasurable early memory of food because of the importance of my father's strong belief in me. He praised and encouraged me, and I always felt safe and secure around him. During the years of my enslavement to food, whenever I felt insecure or fearful, and especially when I had been rejected in a search for intimacy, I turned to mashed potatoes to nurture and soothe myself, and I always held each bite in my mouth for a while to get that little extra dose of comfort.

There are a lot of people in this world who use food as a substitute for security, love, and intimacy. Like Jenny, I experienced the loss of appetite for living and feared the risks of getting wounded that always come when trying to get close to other people. Because my ability to experience life had numbed (in my case as a reaction to sexual abuse as a child), I turned to food for love. Food became the most important thing in my life; all other experiences paled in comparison because nothing made me feel as good as eating did. My need for food became intensified. It became everything. However, constant eating dulled my body further, and slowly all other avenues for experiencing feeling shut down because nothing worked as well as food.

Of all the experiences available to us, eating is one of the few that allow us to employ all of our senses: We taste and smell the food, appreciate its color and attractive preparation, feel its texture as we put it in our mouths and swallow, even hear the bacon sizzling or the crunch of an apple. Both our mind and our body are involved; eating is both an internal and external sensory experience. It is also the one most directly related to our earliest and most urgent needs. One of the first responses we learned as children was "my body feels empty, I'm hungry, I need food." Also, eating is safe; it can be done alone, without risking rejection. It's no wonder that many people turn to food to experience heightened pleasure.

Turning to food for love even works for a while. There is a time, mainly in the anticipation phase or in those first few highly sensitized bites, when the food addict feels whole, alive, and fully in the world.

However, it is a false sensation and a false connection, and the more we turn to food for emotional nurturing, the more disconnected we become and the more starved for life.

Eventually our depression becomes so great that our ability to experience joy through all our senses is significantly diminished. Colors become dull, skin becomes numb, music ceases to thrill, sexual feelings go into limbo. Then one day even food doesn't make us feel better, and we undergo an overall sensory shutdown. We become detached, disconnected, apathetic, alienated, and, above all, depressed. I have been in that state myself, and while I was in it, I saw no way out. Sensory shutdown is one of the most commonly diagnosed symptoms of my incoming patients, and they can't even describe their feelings because they are numb.

For food addicts, eating fulfills all sorts of needs, least of them nutritional. In a risky world, we attempt to satisfy our cravings for nurturance and intimacy with safe, predictable, dependable, emotionally charged food. Our feelings, frozen in other areas, become overly sensitized to experience the many pleasures food has to offer. The most steadfast object of our affection and our most dependable source of comfort becomes not people, but food. Meals become the highlight of the day.

Sexualizing with Food

Whenever I talk to a group and ask them, "Can you relate to sexualizing with food?" immediately their faces brighten. They know exactly what I mean, and hands are up all around the room. I have heard the most amazing things, for example, "I'd rather

12

have a hot dog any day than sex with my husband. I get more satisfaction.'' Many give vivid sensory descriptions of what food means to them. As they talk, their eyes glaze over with a look of rapture and their entire being changes. They have put themselves into a trance merely by describing how they feel about eating. They are sexualizing with food.

Lots of people get pleasure out of eating, but those who sexualize with food have a goal of heightened intensity, like Peggy:

> My passion is for Brach's Chocolate-Covered Cherries. I have a ritual with them: First I bite through the chocolate with a soft little crunch, and then I wait for the cream to squirt and that sweet, wonderful filling to be released on my tongue. I swallow it and then suck on the cherry for a while before I bite into it just a little bit, enough so the juice squirts out. And then I mash the cherry with the chocolate and swallow it real slow. Three of those and I am in heaven. They're better than sex and safer, too.

While Peggy's relationship to food is openly sexual, George's is more romantic. He is a middle-aged man who has been gaining and losing the same one hundred pounds for twenty years. George describes his favorite food in a kind of poetic reverie, as if it were not a sandwich, but a lover:

> What I remember best from my childhood is a pastrami sandwich I used to get on Seventh Avenue around Fiftieth Street in Manhattan. It was a kosher-style delicatessen (and I stress the word *style*) run by an Italian family. The pastrami was cut exceptionally thick, yet it fell apart in your mouth. It was real lean pastrami, and all around the edges were crushed peppercorns. The sandwich was so flavorful you didn't

even need mustard. And if that wasn't enough to send me straight to heaven, the bread was not the usual dry rye, but garlic bread! Wonderful soft little loaves of it, split in half and spread with tasty, buttery garlic. Mmm, what a sandwich. What a pity they went out of business. I still dream about that pastrami on garlic bread.

Another example of this complicated passion for food can be seen in that wonderful movie *Fatso,* in which Dom DeLuise can't resist stopping in the kitchen at his cousin's wake to taste the tomato sauce. The vision of his dreamy eyes cast heavenward while savoring the sauce, as his relatives weep loudly in the other room, reveals better than the most eloquently spoken words how passionately involved people can get with food.

One of the common bonds of food addicts is this intense pleasure they associate with food. Yet it is rarely spoken about. I find it interesting that people think nothing of talking openly about sex, but they would rather not talk about what, when, or how much they eat or what they weigh. Sexual practices may be openly discussed, but our true relationship to food is still a secret. It is the last taboo.

However, not every food addict has such a sexualized relationship with food. In fact, the entire gamut of emotional needs is run: Angry people are attracted to crunchy, chewy food, which they crush and grind with their teeth to express their unspoken feelings. Others seek intimacy with soft, milky foods that provide them with feelings of security and comfort in an emotionally charged way, as I did for years with mashed potatoes and Jenny did with pudding. For Jenny, pudding is literally swirled with emotions. It is a substitute for a missing father and an undemonstrative mother's inability to give affectionate hugs and reassurances. Jenny also used the pudding to swallow her real feelings of loneliness, so she could maintain a cheerful facade and not upset her mother and father.

Although the range of buried emotions expressed with food is wide and full of nuances, they all have one thing in common: heightened feeling. As one patient described her love for strong carbonated drinks: "I like them because they explode on my taste buds. They're a blast-off in my mouth." The strangest part of this intensity is that most often it comes not in the actual eating but in the *anticipation* of eating. When the dessert cart is rolled close to the table, everybody present focuses on the choices and the collective mood begins to elevate. As people ooh and ahh over the sweets, the energy gets bouncy and excitable. Often the dessert cart becomes the emotional highlight of the meal, but the dessert itself rarely lives up to expectations. It's not the eating, it's the foreplay, the thoughts we have in our minds and what we say about the dessert that gives the anticipation phase that special energy.

The same response to the anticipation phase can be seen in other kinds of addictions, like gambling. On the drive to Atlantic City, all the gamblers on the bus are high on thinking and talking about the winnings they anticipate. Like the appearance of the dessert cart, the drive to the casino is usually the most exciting part of the whole experience. The actual dropping of the quarters into the slot machine or the finishing off of that too sweet and slightly gooey piece of cake is secondary. The intensity is around what that food is going to give us. To the food addict, food is more than just food, it's the source of our most heightened emotions.

Sensory Aversions

Not all the sensory distortion is pleasurable. Equally as intense as the passions we have for some foods are the aversions we have for others. It's not what people remember about an unhappy or traumatizing experience, it's what they don't remember that causes the stress. People become numb about what is really bothering them and transfer their bad feelings to a smell, taste, texture, image, or sound associated with the experience, each sensory detail bound up with a feeling of powerlessness they cannot explain or comprehend. These aversions can be clues to the presence of repressed deep feelings. One woman I talked to about aversions responded by putting together for the first time her strong dislike of the color combination yellow and brown and the loss of her mother when she was thirteen years old. Her mother had cultivated iris beds. Unattended in the years following her death, all the delicate colors of the hybrid flowers reverted to yellow and brown. Even today, those colors bring up strong, unexpressed feelings of grief and abandonment she experienced following her mother's death in a car collision.

I developed an aversion to certain foods I associated with my grandfather, who repeatedly sexually abused me as a child. I needed to get rid of the bad feelings I had for what he did, but I still loved him in spite of the abuse. I resolved this terrible dilemma by developing aversions, not to my grandfather (for those feelings would have overpowered me), but toward food I associated with him.

For instance, I have never had a cup of coffee, and I'm not fond of chocolate. As I was writing this book, I put together for the first time those aversions and my grandfather's abuse. I suddenly remembered that there was a chocolate factory in my grandfather's neighborhood, and its smell was always in the air. Chocolate is made with a roasted cocoa bean, which also smells like coffee. I transferred my dread of his innuendoes to an aversion for the odor of chocolate and coffee.

My aversion to turkey is even stronger, perhaps because it relates to the actual abuse. During the holidays I always slept over at my grandparents' house, and my grandfather and I would get up in the middle of the night to baste the turkey. Then, while my grandmother slept in the same bed, he'd fondle me. My repulsion for what he did went into the food he loved. More than thirty years later, I won't touch white turkey meat because he was so fond of it.

These aversions I had for certain smells and tastes affected me physically. They made me feel repulsed and uncomfortable. It was impossible to understand why they would suddenly make me feel so bad. I started thinking I might be crazy. Why should passing by the coffee grinder in the A & P suddenly make me feel so anxious? It's said that smell is the most primal of our senses and that its emotional imprint is the deepest. In my case, smell was the sensory channel through which I experienced my strongest repressed aversions to the abuse.

Sometimes both passions and aversions are present in a single food, as in the way I feel about potatoes. Boiled and left whole the way my grandfather liked them, they represent his abuse, and I hate them, but mashed, they are my father and represent love, safety, and reassurance. I used to get an enormous amount of satisfaction from the fact that my dad hated boiled potatoes also, and I loved the way he used the side of his fork to slice through the potatoes, reducing each big sodden lump to a delicious mass.

During my adolescence, my father had constant high praise for me, which he repeated many times. He was as different a man from my grandfather as it was possible to be—responsible, loyal, and respectful. He never ridiculed me or made me feel uncomfortable about my body and was always expressing his delight at how I was growing into a woman who was attractive, smart, and could have anything I wanted if I set my mind to it. What I really needed to internalize was the message he had given me, not the potatoes! However, I couldn't absorb inspirational messages then. What should have been straight and simple became twisted and obscure because of my grandfather's abuse. I always felt tainted, less than or just not enough.

As I followed the zigzag path of these passions and aversions, I became aware of something very interesting: The feelings associated with the past are invariably triggered in the present by something sensory—a sight, a smell, a taste. It was as if my sense organs, through which I experienced the world, had become disconnected by the trauma of sexual abuse and in the reconnecting made strange. Instead of simply tasting mashed potatoes, I heard my father's praise; I didn't just smell coffee, I felt the unworthiness caused by my grandfather's abuse.

Full of Feeling, Unable to Express, Full of Expression, Unable to Feel

For ten years I went to diet doctors; I weighed as much as 350 pounds and at times was diagnosed as "morbidly obese." It amazes me that all during that time, none of those doctors ever asked, "Is something bothering you?" If a doctor had asked me that, I probably would have burst into tears on the spot. Instead, they talked to me about nutrition, portion control, diet plans, and even surgery, but my weight was a way I was unconsciously expressing myself. All that fat was a clue to what was really bothering me. It was about the abuse. It was an attempt on the part of my body, which always tells the truth, to express my secret—how much that abuse bothered me. If I could have found the words, I would have told all those doctors I went to, "If you want to see my abuse, all I have to do is take off my clothes." However, I couldn't have found the words then because I was in the dark about who I really was. I lacked the solid identity I have now. No one, including myself, was able to guess what my body was trying so hard to express—that I was afraid and hurting deep down inside. Instead, I took my inability to control how much I ate as a message that I was lacking strength or willpower and added it to my base of shame.

Everywhere I go I see people using food to express their repressed emotional needs. Many are expressing a need for protection. Food in the form of layers of fat becomes a fortress that literally keeps others from getting too close, so they'll never risk being hurt by someone. Because I had been introduced to sex before I was ready, it remained something foreign, unpleasant, and even terrifying, so I used food to protect myself from it, thinking that the fat made me less desirable. I also used food to protect myself from my own sexuality, which I experienced as a tiger inside of me that I couldn't control. Because my experience of sex at an early age had been out of my control, my sexuality as an adult continued to feel that way. The more weight I carried, the more protected I felt. No matter how much weight I put on to keep this tiger down, however, I never felt completely safe because strong feelings could suddenly emerge and overwhelm me.

Using food to express a repressed need for protection is common among survivors of sexual abuse. Others may use it to express a repressed need for intimacy, like Jenny and her fondness for prepackaged pudding. However, weight gain only complicates this need for closeness. Often, overeaters are so ashamed of their bodies that they will not allow anyone to be near them; they are so uncomfortable with their bodies that they won't allow sex to be a part of their lives. I remember from the days when I weighed 350 pounds how I didn't want to be touched and that other people didn't want to touch me.

Because of not touching others or being touched, I developed an intense skin hunger and a yearning for physical contact. Feeling vulnerable most of the time, I stayed stuck and too afraid of rejection to take a risk. On the other hand, a plate of mashed potatoes, with its little puddle of butter in the middle, was safe, dependable comfort I could turn to any time I wanted with no risk involved and no surprises.

Disconnection from the 60 Percent

Some people don't even know they have a secret; they just have a numb and gnawing sense of emptiness that won't leave them, or they remain in a state of obsession over food, alcohol, work, relationships, or whatever they choose that gives them a false sense of good feeling so they can function. Or they are unable to accomplish what they really want in life. Most discomforting of all is the feeling of disconnection and enervation. This lack of feeling is the result of a disconnection from their spirit, the 60 percent of themselves that goes by many names, that can't be seen, felt, or heard—their life force, their essence, their God Self.

Regardless of the cause—from a single event, like a death of a parent or a traumatic accident, or from an ongoing situation, like battering, or sexual abuse, or just an insufficient amount of nurturing—disconnection from 60 percent of ourselves is a profound loss. No wonder it renders people barely able to exist in life, let alone enjoy it.

Infants are good examples of connectedness to the 60 percent. Short on verbal skills and barely in control of their muscles, they nevertheless communicate with a powerful impact. They react to stimuli with excitement in every part of their being. When they laugh, their entire bodies laugh; they quiver with life. Just being around their energy amazes me, and I feel more alive in their presence. Infants express the spirit in all its purity, free of negative messages. Becoming disconnected from such a vital part of ourselves is a tragedy. We're left numb and groping in the dark, and our energy is misused to protect or defend ourselves rather than enjoy life.

In childhood, whether disconnection comes quietly or with violence, suddenly or over a period of time, it results in a multiple shattering of the child's core being that has a profound impact on the mature person.

Shattered Identity

As a child, my identity was shattered by sexual abuse. I went from being an outgoing, exuberant, and confident little kid to a guarded, careful one who kept her thoughts to herself, was overly concerned about the well-being of others, and would not take risks for fear of not being accepted. Any time there was a choosing of teammates to play red light, green light or stickball, I was always concerned about being picked even though I was a good athlete, because I believed I was tainted.

To compensate for being unacceptable, I became a doer. I was always striving to feel good about doing *something* because I didn't feel good about being me. However, it couldn't just be doing, it had to be excelling; I was overly conscientious about everything I did. If others practiced a sport or studied a subject for two hours, I put in five. I overdid to cover up my secret that I was tainted, and all my energy went into performing until I was exhausted. I kept to a narrow course and took no risks. As a little kid I was unafraid. I ventured out into the world at an early age, unlike many on my Brooklyn block. When I was five or six, I could take the wrong bus and get help from the right adult to get home again and it was no big deal. I trusted my ability to find someone who would help a cute and bright little kid who was lost.

Because of the disconnection, that confident little kid went into hiding, and I was too afraid of disclosing my secret about my unacceptability to take even the slightest risk. I participated in activities I knew I could excel in. I wouldn't step out into the unknown, because if I failed just once, then Pandora's box would be opened and I wouldn't be accepted. My secret became my identity—I could fool everyone with my good deeds, but deep down I knew that I had no value and was full of shame.

No matter what role we may assume as the result of a shattered identity, it is still a role. Deep down, I used to feel somehow inauthentic, as if I were two people, one with private thoughts and feelings and another who lied to the world. I could never feel comfortable because I always felt I was covering something up. Sometimes I think addicts isolate themselves because they become so tired of playing their role that only by being alone do they get any peace of mind.

When you play roles, you are living in the 30 percent, your cognitive self that tries to figure everything out, that ingenious mind of yours, full of tricks and disguises. As long as we wear the mask we have chosen to defend or protect ourselves from harm, we will achieve only a third of our potential, for our spirit can't dwell in the 30 percent. It is too constricted and an uncomfortable place. In the shattering of identity that comes with a disconnection, the spirit loses its home, and that loss is continuously felt as an inability to experience the feeling of being "at home" in yourself.

Shattered Perception: Becoming Shame Based

Recently I had the luxury of going to a spa, the European kind where women and men are segregated and it is acceptable to walk around wearing nothing at all. I found the experience very telling about how women feel about their bodies. Most of us wore robes, or when briefly naked, we held our bodies in a closed position, trying to conceal our private parts as best we could, avoiding eye contact.

However, a few women walked around nude and proud as statues. Their heads were held high, their shoulders were back, they made no attempt to conceal any part of their bodies, and they looked you square in the eye. They literally had nothing to hide and seemed unconcerned about how others were judging the way they looked. One very heavy older woman walked about totally naked and majestic as if she were a beauty queen.

It became clear to me then that the way women perceived their bodies had nothing to do with what they actually looked like. I was struck by the few women who did walk about nude without concern. They were like Eve before the first bite of that apple. Theirs was the natural state, I thought, the way the rest of us could have felt about our bodies had our self-perception not been shattered by sexual abuse or other attacks on our well-being. Movies and television bombard us with messages that affect our self-perception and make us feel ashamed and unacceptable.

Shame is deep-seated. People can feel guilty about a mistake or a transgression, and once they acknowledge that guilt, they are free of it. However, you are never free of shame. It clings like tar and must be consciously scrubbed away. Shame is the perception of our core identity as worthless. Once these messages penetrate our identity, what we did becomes who we are, and we become shame based. This distorted perception is what makes us feel crazy and dysfunctional. We can't experience ourselves as who we really are, and we can't experience other people.

Sexual Abuse and Shame

Sexual abuse of a child is an act of terror that tragically distorts the self-perception of the victim. Along with the suppression of the actual abuse, I took in the message that there was something wrong with me that caused my grandfather not to value me, and kept that message a secret, too. Internalized, my secret turned into shame. Instead of believing that something wrong was done to me, I believed I had done something wrong. Eventually my perception took another distorted twist, from believing I had done something wrong to believing *I* was wrong. The secret I was keeping became not so much about what happened but about my shame. It had become the core of my identity.

Shattered Trust

A child's trust is very generous. It is their natural state to trust the ones they are close to and from whom they receive love. When that trust becomes shattered, they are put into a twilight zone of confusion. The distorted thinking that results is to universalize the lack of trust. As an adult, because I couldn't trust my grandfather I couldn't trust any man. The very ones I should have been the closest to—my father, my brother—I had dubious relationships with. I felt terrorized around them for no reason. It was with men I loved a lot that I would start to feel the terror. I actually felt safer with men I didn't love; there was no terror with them.

It doesn't take a trauma to have a shattering of

trust. When Jenny was casually told of her parents' separation, her perception of the world as idyllic and unchanging was shattered because the source of the shattering was her parents, the two people who meant the most to her in the world. She also lost her ability to trust. Having experienced how her life could be so completely changed in one moment, she began to believe that at any minute, when she least expected it, her world could blow up in her face. By internalizing this message, her ability to trust was frozen, and Jenny had trouble making the most casual connection. The risk was just too great.

Distorted Values

The value we give ourselves reflects the way we were valued by people we were closest to as children. If any of those relationships get distorted for any reason, it can distort every future relationship. As time goes by, those values turn into long-term beliefs about the way life should be, the way family relationships should be, and about the world in general.

We also absorb values from other powerful sources such as television, movies, magazines, and popular music. These learned values can also distort perception of the self, for their message is that only if you buy something, go somewhere, or do something will your life have meaning. If you pick up on these distorted values, you're bound to perceive yourself as inadequate.

We are bombarded with messages all the time. If you don't have a clear knowledge of who you are, if you don't feel your life has meaning or purpose, if you don't know what you believe in—if you're disconnected from your spirit—it is very easy to internalize those values. When you are finally reconnected, you will discover the Real You and determine your own values.

Trauma and Disconnection

Since the Vietnam War, the long-term effects of trauma on civilians as well as veterans has been widely studied.

Many families have a member who came back from war suffering from what used to be called "shell shock" but is now called post-traumatic stress disorder, or PTSD. Decades later, these veterans may continue to function marginally and never return to their old selves. They often still relive their war experiences in their sleep. Part of them didn't come home from the war, and that part was their spirit. Usually these vets won't talk about what happened to them in the war. It becomes a secret that becomes more of a burden to keep buried as time goes by.

It has been found that the brain is permanently altered by even a single traumatic experience. One of the symptoms is memory loss. The traumatizing event itself is often completely repressed, and the person may have amnesia about events surrounding it as well. Of course, nothing is forgotten. All the feelings that were too much to cope with at the time of the trauma are buried to become bothersome years later.

People who experience trauma often bury the experience and the feelings generated from it in order to "get on with life." However, in their disconnected state, these feelings manifest themselves in unhealthy ways, they lose the greatest part of themselves, and the secret is still there sabotaging their life.

Many people are unaware they are holding secrets. They only know that they feel empty and disconnected. If you are wondering whether you are holding a secret in the form of unexpressed, repressed deep feelings, take the following quiz.

QUIZ: Do You Have a Secret?

To each of the following twenty-five statements, give a score that most nearly describes yourself:

4 Nearly all the time. You definitely identify with the statement to the extent that the behavior or feeling it describes has become a problem in getting what you want out of life.

3 Often. You identify with the statement, but the problem could be worse.

2 Some of the time. Although you identify, the feeling or behavior does not cause major problems in your life.

1 Rarely, if ever. You do not identify with the statement, or if you do, it is a unique occurrence, or it used to be true but is no longer.

_____ 1. I feel stuck, as if I just can't get my life going.

_____ 2. I do not voice my true feelings and thoughts to others.

_____ 3. I feel inauthentic, an outsider, as if I didn't belong.

_____ 4. I binge in secret.

_____ 5. I tell lies about insignificant things for no reason.

_____ 6. I mentally rehearse what I will say in confrontations with others but avoid actually confronting them.

_____ 7. I feel as if I am not important, that my opinions and feelings don't count.

_____ 8. I don't feel entitled to feel as good as I do.

_____ 9. I have strong aversions to certain people and/or foods.

_____10. I have strong aversions to a certain color, sound, texture, taste, or smell.

_____11. I have trouble remembering things that have happened to me in my life.

_____12. There is a destructive pattern to my relationships.

_____13. I have dreams of being chased or falling or dreams where there are words written on signs or on a page or in which there are objects that have a symbolic personal meaning.

_____14. I don't trust myself.

_____15. I feel as if there is something missing in my life.

_____16. I have a numbness in my body.

_____17. I have pains in my body that doctors are unable to diagnose.

_____18. I feel lonely even when people are around.

_____19. There are taboo subjects in my family. People, events, or certain topics like sex are

29

not talked about or are only implied with a strongly judgmental attitude.

_____20. People have told me I talk angrily or fearfully in my sleep.

_____21. There are things I do in secret that I don't want anyone to know about.

_____22. I feel a lot of shame for no reason.

_____23. I have a limited ability to experience sexual pleasure.

_____24. I have favorite foods I binge on when I have unmet emotional needs.

_____25. I have a problem with addictive compulsions.

SCORING

1–25. Generally, people in this range are successful in meeting goals, open, satisfied with their lives, and secure, or they may be in denial. If you scored in this low range and still feel bad about yourself, this book will help dissolve your defenses so you can get to what's really bothering you.

25–50. It is likely that you have some issues that have not been completely worked through.

50–75. It is likely that you have repressed memories or unfinished business that is giving you problems.

75–100. You have a secret that is giving you a lot of discomfort, and you are trying to seek relief. This book can help you.

Becoming Frozen

Another symptom of PTSD is a prolonged state of emotional and physical numbness. When small animals are overwhelmed, they freeze, or "play possum" by appearing to be dead or asleep. Children react in a similar way to a trauma, and part of them stays frozen long after the danger is past. In an adult, the part that is still frozen is expressed by zoning out, lowered sensory response, and a need to be in a chemically altered state to get in touch with feelings.

I became a frozen child; the part of me that remained frozen had to do with feelings about my sexuality. During the turbulence of adolescence, when the body metamorphoses into a sexual being and new and exciting feelings emerge, my body felt nothing. It remained frozen by the trauma of sexual abuse. Because of what my grandfather did to me, I perceived sex as something bad and wrong, and so I shut down my sexual feelings. Even in marriage, although able to enjoy sex to a certain degree because it was now legal and condoned by God, I still remained mostly numb and detached. Many nights after having sex I would go to the kitchen and eat, trying to comfort myself with something I could feel, smell, and taste. Somehow my adult sex life remained tainted by the childhood abuse.

Dissociation

Another symptom of PTSD that contributes to this feeling of numbness is the tendency to leave the body, or to dissociate. I became detached from my body because of my great confusion over the bind I was in with my grandfather. On the one hand, I was dependent on him, loved him, and loved all the attention he lavished on me. On the other hand, he abused me. When I could not reconcile the good side of my grandfather with the bad side, part of me detached. While he fondled me, I "left" my body. I have no idea where I went when I left my body, I just don't remember being there. Yet I can still recall every detail of the room in which the abuse happened. I can tell you the kind of molding around the door, I can see the false window between the dining room and the bedroom of my grandparents' railroad apartment, I can see the clock on the wall, I can see everything in that bedroom from the perspective of me on the bed. It's almost as if I went into the woodwork. By focusing on my surroundings, I fled my body through my eyes and concentrated not on what was happening, but on what I was seeing. In that way, I managed to rescue my sanity.

Out-of-body experiences are another form of dissociation. People remember the event as happening but as if they were a witness to the scene, from a point of view outside the body. A middle-aged man retained the memory of his mother battering him as a child, but he remembered it as a visualization of himself sitting on the stairs and observing the beating. For years he was convinced the abuse was actually happening to his older brother. Dissociation is a form of mental cauterizing, a protective emergency measure that prevents an escape into insanity. It is a highly creative flight from pain.

Another form of dissociation is the split personality. Whereas people like me escape into the woodwork, multiples escape into another personality. That way they don't have to experience what's going on. A famous case is Sybil, who was sexually tortured by her mother. Sybil became a multiple personality, developing many personae before she began to integrate them. Developing multiple personalities is an extreme form of dissociation, but it shows how far our 30 percent will go to protect our being.

Regardless of what defenses are employed, for all who experience a trauma, the same journey of integration needs to take place. The body, mind, emotions, and spirit must be reconnected to develop our core beings and become whole and healthy.

QUIZ: Traumalogue

Symptoms of the long-term effects of a trauma are reflected in the following thirty-four questions. To each statement, give a score that most nearly describes yourself:

4 Nearly all the time. You identify with the statement to the extent that the behavior or feeling it describes has become a problem in getting what you want out of life.

3 Often. You identify with the statement, but the problem could be worse.

2 Some of the time. Although you identify, the feeling or behavior does not cause major problems in your life.

1 Rarely, if ever. You do not identify with the statement, or if you do, it is a unique occurrence, or it used to be true but is no longer.

_____ 1. I feel crazy, unique, or different.

_____ 2. I fear sleeping alone or being alone in the dark.

_____ 3. I feel guilty, shameful, or marked.

_____ 4. I am attracted to people who abuse me.

_____ 5. I feel numb or distant from my body.

_____ 6. I have nightmares and night terrors.

_____ 7. I feel trapped.

_____ 8. I am not at home in my own body.

_____ 9. I am self-destructive and self-abusive.

_____ 10. I use food, alcohol, and/or drugs compulsively.

_____ 11. I cry but don't know what I'm upset about.

_____ 12. I feel impulsive, like a child.

_____ 13. I don't recognize my own anger.

_____ 14. I wear a lot of clothes, even in warm weather.

_____ 15. I gag or have trouble swallowing.

_____ 16. I start fires or steal.

_____ 17. I am particular about having privacy.

_____ 18. I fear losing control.

_____ 19. I really don't care whether I live or die.

_____ 20. I hurt myself on purpose.

_____ 21. I don't feel sexual desire.

_____ 22. I find it difficult to be close in nonsexual ways.

_____ 23. I don't remember much about my childhood.

_____ 24. I'm compulsively seductive or asexual.

_____ 25. I'm afraid of being abusive.

_____ 26. My family invalidates my feelings.

_____ 27. I minimalize: "It wasn't that bad."

_____ 28. I trust too much or too little.

_____ 29. I have abused or neglected my children.

_____30. People take advantage of me in relationships.

_____31. I have attempted suicide.

_____32. I can't tell one feeling from another.

_____33. I feel enraged.

_____34. I think of my childhood as being perfect.

SCORING

0–34. You have strong recovery, or you are fortunate in that you have not had a traumatizing experience.

34–68. It is unlikely that you have buried feelings around a trauma because your scoring does not reflect the most observable symptoms of its long-term effects.

68–102. Something happened to you that has resulted in a disconnection. Whether it is of traumatic or non-traumatic nature it is impossible to determine at this point.

102–136. You are in a lot of pain. This book can help you.

There Doesn't Have to Be a Trauma

The problem with the word *trauma* is it evokes something dramatic and violent, but that isn't always the case. It's important to remember that it's not an event that traumatizes, it's what happens to the spirit. Any time there is a repression of unacceptable, unexpressed feelings, there is an impact on your core identity. Jenny experienced the divorce of her parents as a shattering event even though her parents were so civilized they didn't so much as raise their voices in anger. Nevertheless, the disconnection from Jenny's spirit was as complete as if she had undergone an act of violence.

Disconnection can take place for a wide variety of reasons. It often occurs in children whose parents are emotionally immature. These children are neglected in deeply damaging but hidden ways, for the parents are too busy focusing on themselves to really attend to their children's needs. Or the parents may go through the motions of taking good care of their children, but they can't see them as separate beings. Rather, they perceive their children as little extensions of themselves. Such parents manipulate and usurp the child's right to define him- or herself. "This is my little doctor/scientist/dancer," they say as a way of introduction, marking the child with the future profession of their choice (which often involves thwarted dreams of their own). Meanwhile, the children are denied the freedom of forming their own identity and must later struggle to attain their own sense of self.

Receiving strong negative messages about sexuality from parents or other authority figures can also cause a loss of spirit just as much as a physical act of abuse. I am always amazed at how many obese people there are in the congregations of strict religious groups. The concept of original sin and of sexuality as something dirty and to be feared is often overlooked as causing an impact on our spirit. People who internalize these negative messages don't understand that our sexuality is a gift from God. Instead, every time they have sex they feel dirty. They feel guilty for having sexual feelings and thus cut themselves off from that part of their being.

36

Also frequently overlooked as a cause of disconnection is bonding with someone who was disconnected. Jenny identified strongly with her mother and came away with feelings of low desirability and self-esteem because that's the way her mother felt about herself. Because I really loved my mother, who was also sexually abused by my grandfather—her father—I took on her beliefs about men and sexuality. Sometimes she didn't have to say a word. I felt her negative energy about men and knew something was wrong but couldn't understand exactly what it was. My mom had difficulty trusting men and had a tendency to isolate herself from them. I was closely bonded with her, so I also distanced myself from men.

A basic lack of communication exists in many dysfunctional families, and this, too, can end up quietly shattering the spirit. People in these families never learn to express who they are or what they want. They grow up feeling isolated even when together. When they go out in the world and try to have a life of their own, they feel rootless, as if there is no place where they really belong because they never learned to define themselves as who they really are.

Cultural influences can also cause us to lose spirit. The nuclear family, once the norm, is rapidly becoming extinct, and family as a strong base of security and support does not exist for many. Nor have alternative support systems developed for them. Divorce and the scattering of extended families are so common they are often overlooked as deep underlying causes of many people's disconnection. A social order that used to be mutually sustained and nourished—parents, grandparents, children, aunts, uncles, and cousins, plus long-term friends and neighbors—now has a 50 percent chance of being a single-parent household. With the scattering of the extended family and the shattering of the nuclear family, no wonder so many people feel so lost!

Family ties are no longer strengthened by personal histories passed on from generation to generation. Brothers and sisters live in the same town and hardly talk to each other, or if they do get together, it's around the diversion of a video screen. When a culture lacks identity and the traditional family is a thing of the past, we lose our sense of history, our roots, and our values. In the social and cultural void, we relate to food or other substances or relationships—anything to give us a feeling of belonging, connectedness, and well-being—even if just temporarily.

Added to the growing list of nontraumatic causes for a disconnection is yet another new phenomenon in our history—the constant bombardment of destructive messages about our bodies from all forms of the advertising media. Visuals pack an especially powerful wallop. The underlying message these ads repeat is, "You're not enough. You could look better. You don't smell right. Buy something." Women live with an especially heavy burden of enculturation that tells them they must be not only forever thin and beautiful, but forever young or they lose their desirability.

With that kind of media warfare being waged against our self-image, you could have grown up with saintly parents and the best of families, had the gentlest and most humanistic of religious upbringings, and still feel horrible about your body. Managing *not* to take in these harmful media messages about yourself would be something of a miracle!

For whatever nontraumatic reason people become disconnected, the end result is the same as for the traumatized: They feel inferior and not enough just the way they are. However, the nontraumatized have a special burden. They wonder why they are so sensitive over what they may believe is comparatively little to complain about. That can make them even more stuck than the traumatized. I often think these people have a little more difficulty healing themselves because there isn't an awful event to point to and say, "See? This is the cause of my depression." In treatment they often have a hard time comparing their mostly uneventful childhoods to the horror stories they hear from survivors of trauma and abuse. One patient described himself as "just mildly neurotic, but hopelessly fucked up." Nevertheless, they are just as disconnected and exist in the same anxiety bath as do survivors of trauma. They assume the same defensive patterns and also hate their bodies. They have all lost their appetite for living and feel as if their lives aren't going anywhere.

It's the Secrets That Keep You Stuck

For years I have been intrigued by the connections between food and sex, food and intimacy, and food and love. Food becomes a trigger for some of our most intense emotions. We invest food with such strong feelings and turn to it to fulfill our deepest needs. I am now convinced that the power we give to food is really about our secrets. Instead of constantly being on a quest to discover a new diet, we need to be on a quest to discover our secrets, the ones that may be buried so deeply they are even hidden from ourselves. Some people do such a good job of denying that they don't even know that they have a secret. All they have is a numb and gnawing sense of emptiness that year after year won't leave them. They remain in a state of obsessing over food, alcohol, work, relationships, or whatever they choose to use that gives them a false sense of well-being, so they can just keep going. Or they are unable to accomplish what they really want to out of life.

Why is it that some people get over sad things that happen to them in their childhood and others stay stuck? I have become convinced that it is more than what happened to them (because people are so remarkably resilient and can recover from the most traumatic events); it's the secrets that keep them stuck, self-absorbed, and unable to move forward.

Whatever it is that has been forgotten, numbed, or suppressed must be dredged up before we can get on with the challenge of living, for these deep, unexpressed feelings that have been buried are twisted and hurtful in the way they are expressed today. They have become unconscious self-destructive messages that we will unwittingly repeat until we consciously reframe them.

That quest to find our buried secrets is the goal of Chapter II of this book: to examine the clues that will lead us to those unresolved issues (and believe me, we wouldn't be human if we didn't have them) and to release the feelings that were suppressed at the time. Because long-kept secrets are so well hidden, the only map we have is subtle and blurred. Paths that should be straight are crooked, and there are many blind alleys, but the clues are there. Our behavior is one, but we have to look beyond all the disguises we wear to protect our secret. Sensory clues are another indication of something hidden, as are strange and twisted connections in our relationships with both people and food. As we become accustomed to searching our past and present behavior for clues, we may also discover patterns—repeated self-destructive behavior, most readily seen in our love choices—which may have had grave consequences in our lives.

"Seek and ye shall find," the Bible says. I know in my heart that if you embark on this treasure hunt with me in search of your disconnected self, you will discover what you need to know about what you have forgotten. Know in your heart that you're God's kid and commend yourself for getting this far in the journey. Believe me, it's a beginning to a wonderful life.

Because feeling stuck is so much a part of holding a secret, know that putting off making a decision to continue on this journey is a decision not to make a decision. But let me ask you this: when will it be time for you? Taking the first step today will begin the reconnection process so that one day your spirit, well nourished and fully charged, can propel you forward to fulfill your greatest, fondest, and most long-held dreams.

ACTIVITIES
Days 1-11

Interspersed throughout this book you will find ninety activities, one for each day of the ninety days. You can skip them entirely or simply read through them, but I can guarantee that reading alone will not result in change. You need to take action if you want that to happen. I recommend you complete the eleven days of activities before going on to read Chapter II.

Doing the activities will require the purchase of a notebook and a few minutes of your time each day of the ninety days. Activity One, Create a Safe Environment, will provide the other essential—a place where you will feel safe enough for your secrets to emerge.

These activities are designed to be done alone, but many require you to change the way you relate to the world and other people. Although they are intended to be a catalyst to accelerate recovery, understand there is no quick fix, and recovery is a process without a timetable. Nevertheless, by making a concentrated effort to complete these activities, you will go a long way in dealing with any secrets you may have and receive a head start on your journey into recovery.

Day 1: Create a Safe Environment

People who don't feel safe won't allow themselves to experience repressed information. The following actions will send a message of protection to the part of you that may not feel safe. You need to coax that part of yourself along.

Think for a moment about the things that make you feel safe—tangibles that make up an environment in which you feel protected. These may include an object you inherited from someone you love, fresh flowers, or certain paintings or photographs that have special meaning. We all carry within us unique and deeply imprinted images of safety. They will come up for you if you give some thought to what specifically helps you. When the images surface, gather these objects and use them to create your special place—an environment where you feel safe and unafraid.

Your safe place should be readily accessible—better in the next room than a walk or a car ride away—but it should also be a place where you can be private—the kind of place where people knock on a door before entering. Maybe it is your bedroom or a part of a room that you can transform into a sanctuary for yourself.

In the safe place you have created, you will be able to do the activities in this book with a full heart. You are the protector now, and the environment you have created gives evidence of that fact to the part of you that still does not believe. Here you will be able to write journal entries and other forms of memory jogging, to answer the many diagnostic questionnaires, to think and probe and meditate, to take risks and experience old feelings, and to do the ninety activities in this book within the ninety days.

Day 2: What I Remember

Buy a big college-ruled spiral notebook with three to five sections. Label the first section "What I Remember." For each of the following ninety days, record a single memory from your childhood in one sentence and describe the feeling attached to it. Also describe the effect the memory has on you today, if any.

Recently I conducted a group session of "What do you remember?" People sat in a circle and wrote down a one-sentence memory and a feeling attached to it. I was astonished and overwhelmed at how quickly the memories came up and the heights and depths of the emotional response. Along with the bad stuff, wonderfully illuminating moments popped up. One woman remembered being six years old and in love. She and her six-year-old boyfriend made a commitment to love each other forever. Her recollection gave her such joy. Another woman remembered seeing a double rainbow with her dad.

Getting in touch with rainbows and six-year-old declarations of eternal love floods the spirit with a rush of joy. Getting in touch with painful memories, although not joyful, is also cathartic, because we have a tendency to stuff these events away, believing we'll lose control if we remember. It's important to have them stimulated so they can be dislodged and no longer keep us stuck.

Day 3: Safe Keepers

Label the second section of your spiral notebook "Journal." Here you will do a lot of the writing involved in the activity work.

In your journal, make a list of all the people in your life whom you feel safe with—in the past and in the present. If you have photographs of those people, display them in your safe place. If you have things they made or gave you, include those objects and think of them as amulets of protection.

Day 4: Baby's Toys

In your journal, recall a significant toy from your childhood and write about it. If you have a baby book, it can help stimulate your recollection, because it often has a place for birthday and holiday gifts to be recorded. Describe that significant toy. Did it have a name? Why was it significant? Try to find one like it and keep it in your safe place.

Day 5: A Vision for You

Affirmations are statements you say to yourself that change your self-perception, if only for a moment. However, that momentary improvement in the way you think about yourself can be sustained by repetition. By saying these affirmations out loud every day for ninety days, you will begin to internalize messages about how special you really are. Sometimes we lose sight of the truly wonderful things about us; bad feelings overshadow the good. These affirmations will remind you of the good things, and in time these thoughts will transfer over to the way you act, and soon you will see yourself as the wonderful being you are and treat yourself with the love and care you deserve.

Every day in your journal, preferably at bedtime, write down an affirmation by completing the sentence "I am . . ." I think affirmations should be done at bedtime rather than during the day. When we are out and about, we are too into the external world. Writing the affirmations down right before you go to sleep nourishes your spirit.

What you tell yourself you are is crucial to your recovery. Who am I? I am loving, caring, abundant, giving. That's who I really am. It is such a simple statement, but it took many years to discover those four words. Your "I am" statements can be different each day, but in the process they help shape and focus your identity.

Look for energy words that convey loving action and describe how you want to be experienced by others. Every evening, as you make your "I am" statement, your mind has the amazing and mysterious capacity to absorb this image of yourself and create new pathways in your thinking that, together with action, will help you get what you want.

Day 6: Progressive Relaxation

The body can facilitate the releasing of the secrets it is holding through the conscious release of tension. It is recommended that whenever you embark on a discovery, begin by unlocking your muscles. The following exercise is most effective when accompanied by soft and soothing music. Lie comfortably on the floor with a pillow under your head, close your eyes, and slowly progress from one group of muscles to another until your body feels loose and free.

As you tense each group of muscles, hold the tension for about five seconds, and as you slowly release the tension silently say, "Relax and let go." Then take a deep breath, and as you slowly exhale silently repeat the message: "Relax and let go."

The Head

- Wrinkle your forehead.
- Squint your eyes tightly.
- Open your mouth widely.
- Push your tongue against the roof of your mouth.
- Clench your jaw tightly.

The Neck

- Push your head back into the pillow.
- Bring your head forward to touch your chest.
- Roll your head to your right shoulder.
- Roll your head to your left shoulder.

The Shoulders

- Shrug your shoulders up as if to touch your ears.
- Shrug your right shoulder up as if to touch your ear.
- Shrug your left shoulder up as if to touch your ear.

The Arms and Hands

- Hold your arms out and make a fist with each hand.
- One side at a time, push your hands toward the floor.
- One side at a time, make a fist, bend your arm at the elbow, and tighten up your arm while holding the fist.

The Chest and Lungs

- Take a deep breath.
- Tighten the chest muscles.

The Back

- Arch your back.

The Stomach

- Tighten your stomach muscles.
- Push your stomach muscles out.
- Contract your stomach muscles.

The Hips, Legs, and Feet

- Tighten your hips.
- Push the heels of your feet into the floor.
- Tighten your leg muscles below the knee.
- Curl your toes under as if to touch the bottom of your feet.
- Bring your toes up as if to touch your knees.

When you have completely relaxed all these groups of muscles, count from one to three while you move first your feet, then your body, stretch, and open your eyes.

Day 7: Trust Exercise

1. Write down the names of people you know, personally or professionally, in whom you have complete trust. Why do you trust them?
2. Based on your above answer, what does the word *trust* mean to you?
3. Is your name on the list of people you trust? If not, why not?

Day 8: Childhood Ecstasy

In your journal, record the happiest memory of your childhood. Why is it your happiest memory? What specifically do you recall about that day? Describe the other people involved. Compare it to other high moments in your life.

Day 9: Passions and Aversions

In your journal, describe any aversions you may have to a smell, color, texture, sound, or taste. Describe also any unusually strong aversion you may have for an individual.

Now describe your favorite food. How does eating it make you feel? How long has it been your favorite? When is your favorite time to eat it and under what circumstances?

Day 10: Dream Book

Label a third section of your notebook "Dream Book." Leave it open to this section at night by your bed so you can capture those fleeting dreams that seem to evaporate as soon as you are fully awake. Just having the open notebook by your bedside encourages your mind to retain the important clues about your secrets to which your dreams give you access.

For today, record in your dream book any recurring dreams you have. What theme or scenario is repeated? What are the feelings around the dream? If you have no recurring dreams, do you have any that leave an emotional impact on your conscious life, causing you to wake in fear or to feel depressed the next day?

Day 11: What Have You Done to Take Care of Yourself Today?

You will be keeping still another daily record. Each night before going to bed, before or after you write your daily affirmation, note down the things you did that day to take care of yourself. Don't overlook the ordinary things, like matching up all the loose socks in your sock drawer or getting a haircut. Be sure to include the things you couldn't manage to do for yourself before and describe how taking care of yourself makes you feel.

Many people, especially survivors of abuse, have a terrible time valuing themselves, because it runs counter to their deepest convictions. By keeping a record of what you are doing for yourself every day, you will enable yourself to develop a feeling of worth—filling that hollow core with good nourishment. This activity will also encourage you to find ways to care for yourself *today,* if only to have something to record!

As the ninety days go by, you will find so many good ways to take care of yourself that you will begin to present a new face to the world. You may still feel miserable much of the time, but people will begin to react to you differently. You will have changed your behavior even though you have not changed your feelings, and that, my friend, is a great beginning.

II

Discovery

One's own self is well hidden from oneself: of all
mines of treasure, one's own is the last to be dug up.
—Friederich Nietzsche

Following the Crooked Path

In the nursery tale "Hansel and Gretel," two children leave their wicked stepmother and go out into
the woods because there is no food in the house.
Hansel tells Gretel to leave a trail of bread crumbs
so they can find their way back home. This trail of
bread crumbs can be a metaphor for the clues our
inner child's mind retains as a trace memory to guide
the disconnected adult home.

In the process of recovery, we experience the same
difficulty that Hansel and Gretel went through. The
birds ate most of their clues. We bury our memories
so deeply that some are gone forever. For many years
we become lost in the woods, but fortunately, with
the passage of time, the clues that do remain grow in

51

prominence until they all but glow in the dark. In food addicts, for example, the clue literally mushrooms in the form of excess fat as more and more we express our secrets with our bodies.

A Love for the Altered State

One obvious clue is addiction, often developing at the onset of puberty, when confusion over emerging sexuality adds to the confusion about identity. Amid this confusion, people turn to something outside of themselves for relief. We've been encultured into using something outside of ourselves to feel better and to believe in the "fast-easy-quick" approach to temporary relief afforded by addictive substances.

A familiar story shared in recovery is about the intense high we get the first time we drink alcohol or take any mood-changing drug. We continue to speak of that first experience as if it were an epiphany, which for many of us it was—the first time since a disconnection that we experienced our frozen feelings. In the thrall of our addiction, we become the laughing drunks, the crying drunks, the violent drunks, because only while in an altered state do we have access to our emotions. Needing to be high in order to feel is a very big clue to a buried secret.

Disguises

Other clues, more complex but also telling, can be seen in the roles we assume. When we became disconnected from our spirit, we lost our core identity, and we were forced to create a new one, a mask, that we use to present ourselves to others. We play these roles with much conviction because along with trying to convince others this is who we are, we're trying to convince ourselves.

The Counselor

Some people are so busy repressing their feelings they don't even acknowledge the fact that they are depressed. In fact, they can be some of the most cheerful people you know, who not only keep their own spirits up but yours as well. It is the way they learned to cope with depression. They are the first ones to advise you or cheer you on. However, counselors have a false sense of hope; it comes out of their need to cheer themselves up when they feel miserable, which is most of the time.

The Doer

Counselors are all talk; doers are all action. They are "summertime" friends; they are there for everyone when the heat is on and everyone else is on vacation. Doing for others was a role I had assumed early in life as a way to create an identity for myself. I took on the emotional needs of everyone, including my parents. As I grew up, being a doer remained a comfortable role for me to play because it was familiar. I was always on the go, doing whatever it took to meet the needs of others. It was the only way I could feel good about myself: "See, I'm a good person, I help other people." Being overly conscientious is always a source of comfort to shame-based people. Each good deed helps camouflage the awful person we really think we are. After years of frantic doing, what we do *becomes* who we are. It is an attempt to fill that deep and empty void, but deep down, it never does.

As I continued to play the role of doer, I found my energy being dissipated because there was no balance in my relationships. I rarely got back as much as I gave, but I had to keep giving because doing something good for another was the only way I could feel better about myself. For a brief while, I felt untainted.

As long as I stayed busy and continued to do good things with a lot of energy and good will, I could hide my shame and lack of value from the world. I truly believed I had to build an identity, deed by deed, based on accomplishments.

The People Pleaser

People pleasers seem to be doers, but it's not the actual performance of good deeds that gives them satisfaction, but being well liked that provides their identity. They are effusive in their praise, and their promises are many. People pleasers, however, promise more than they can possibly deliver, and they add reneging on those promises to their heavy burden of guilt. People pleasers are so fearful of displeasing anyone that they can't confront a waiter or an airline clerk or even someone in their employ. Their need to be liked takes precedence over everything else, including their own best interests. In such people, the need to be liked has become universalized; it applies to everyone without distinction, from the abusive spouse to the intrusive neighbor to the stranger who just cut in front of them in the movie line.

People pleasers are very generous people. They'll give you their last ten dollars. Their generosity, however, is tainted by doing the right thing for the wrong reason. People pleasers often feel empty, and no matter how good we are, we are never, ever good enough. That feeling is reinforced by the feedback we get from the world. Unfortunately, many people have low self-esteem and tend to lose respect for anyone who would care so much about wanting to please them. Such people are, in fact, suspicious of people pleasers. That response makes the people pleaser so anxious that he or she has to try even harder. The cycle exhausts them so much they rarely have time to actually do anything that pleases themselves.

Even when people pleasers accomplish something great, like writing a two-hundred-page document, all they will be able to focus on is the misspelling on page sixteen. I remember when speaking to a group, I would always focus on the one person who didn't seem pleased. It didn't matter that thousands loved me. I had to convince that one person. The real person I had to convince was myself.

Why do people pleasers act in this often self-defeating way? Because they have been terrorized. Any strongly negative emotional response that becomes universalized is a clue to the presence of a trauma. If you universalize the need to be liked, in that you can't risk offending anyone—not even an insolent stranger whose services you are paying for—without feeling bad about yourself for hours afterward, know that your response fits the PTSD syndrome and that with a lot of nourishment to your spirit you can live without fear. You can stop having to be so pleasing!

The Victim

When you have only one identity, that of a victim, you are totally empty if you let it go. It's fear of that void that makes the victim cling to the role, no matter how inappropriate or even downright dangerous the situation. Chronic victims have a way of framing every situation as one in which they've been taken advantage of, and of course, others will feel sorry for them. Victims confuse this sympathy with acceptance of who they are as a person. Their identity is completely entwined with that of the disguise they wear.

For someone with a secret, playing the role of victim becomes a way of expressing the unknown truth about themselves. "Don't you see? I'm a victim," they are saying. However, just as when I tried to express my abuse with my weight, no one hears or understands.

The Control Freak

Fear is also behind the rigid style of behavior of the control freak. Its purpose is to protect the unsafe and the insecure. Controllers go for perfection and set up every outcome in order to feel safe. They usually justify every action with logic to ensure that you don't see their fear.

In school, controllers have to get A's; anything less and they are devastated. They hate surprises. As adults they must be personally involved in every decision that comes their way—no matter how insignificant—from planning which route to take to whether the sandwiches should be cut in halves or quarters. And if control freaks don't get their way, they go into a tailspin! They usually do end up getting their way because they have a much stronger need than others to control the outcome.

Controllers are also rigid about their food. I received a long-distance call one day from a woman who asked me about protein for a vegetarian. How much? What kind? How often? I couldn't get her to focus on anything but food during the entire conversation, even though at the time she was reading *It's Not What You're Eating, It's What's Eating You*, a book whose premise is that dieting doesn't work. Because she spent all her energy obsessing over *what* she put in her mouth, she couldn't see that her real problem with food was *why* she overate.

The rigidity of the controller is really about the little part that's *not* in control—the feelings of pain, rage, and confusion. Deep down, controllers know there is no such thing as *total* control, and that makes them feel furious and helpless.

The Crusader

Over the years, I have noticed that a high number of survivors of abuse are activists in human and animal rights causes. It's as if they have diverted all their feelings about their own abuse into speaking out about injustices perpetrated upon others. The more vulnerable and helpless the victim, the more intense their fervor. One woman crusader I know described how, from an early age, she had to look on while a younger brother was frequently beaten by a foster parent. She described how helpless she felt (for her interventions only made the beatings worse) and how filled with unexpressed rage she was at what she had witnessed. By the time she was in high school, she was planning to become a missionary. Now she is very active in saving baby seals in the Pacific Northwest. In a way, it is as if she can now intervene and do something. Throwing herself with fervor into a cause to save the helpless is a way to keep the lid on all her repressed feelings.

Like people pleasers, crusaders are held at arm's length by the world at large, which, understandably, doesn't trust their motives. Both groups are intent on forcing others' feelings. They can't just let things happen and be. Whereas people pleasers are putting all their efforts into getting you to like them, crusaders want you to change your opinion or even your beliefs. In both cases, the focus is on their own agenda and not a real intimate connection.

The Dreamer

Neither flight nor fight is an available alternative to the child in the face of danger, but nature has provided an alternative response: escape through the imagination. I am often amazed at how creative the act of dissociation is, maybe because it emanates from the vividness of the child's imagination. In the process of dissociation, children create fantastic dreamworlds, magical places where they have superhuman powers and can even fly and everyone is wonderful, kind, and good. I often wonder how many artists' visions begin in the fantasy world they have dreamed in order to escape from abuse.

I know an incest survivor who is a wonderful painter. She seeks out the beauty of everything that comes into her sight. Take a walk with her and she will point out a hundred things that interest her or give delight. One of a handful of memories she has from childhood became the signature of her life. It is of herself as a child drawing a multipetaled rose in colored chalk on a blackboard and showing it to a kindly relative.

In treatment, my patient realized the memory was a clue to something repressed. That single visual memory of a rose was a clue to the repeated abuse by a stepfather. In order to dissociate from the trauma, she fixated on the floral design of a sofa cover, tracing each leaf and petal. In her creative flight into the rose, she was able to repress all the ugliness of her stepfather's act, leaving in its place only an image of beauty.

However, she had one major problem: Along with the repressed memories went her creative expression. Artistically she was paralyzed, for her sense of self was diminished. She daydreamed through school and was a perpetual underachiever. Until she worked through her trauma, she didn't even think of herself as a creative person. Once she went into recovery, she was able to set her creative spirit free. She hasn't stopped painting since.

Dreamers carry with them into adulthood a facility to put themselves into a trance, to "zone out." They have a way of appearing to listen to you when their minds are a thousand miles away. Their attention span is brief and their memory short. Zoning out becomes habitual until they are just going through the motions of being present. Not only do they not fully participate in life, but other people are unable to experience them.

People with secrets often play more than one of the roles just described, assuming one identity and then another according to the circumstances and even playing more than one role at a time. They go through life like guests at a costume ball: People have to guess who they really are. People with secrets often get stuck in their role-playing for long periods of time because the roles seem to be providing them with the gratification they need. In fact, rarely have I known people to give up a disguise while it's still working for them.

Sometimes the disguises gradually wear away as time passes, and the person stays the same, unable to make the changes life requires for happiness and success: The excellent student continues to stay in his entry-level job, or the free spirit continues to be economically dependent on her parents. Sooner or later, the party is over—the roles we play don't work any more, the money stops coming, the loved one demands a change, or the career goes nowhere. Often the failure is a blessing in disguise because it is after our defenses fail that we become motivated to seek help.

The Delay Factor

The more traumatic the event, the deeper it is buried. In the case of incest, statistics show that most survivors don't begin coming to grips with the issue of their childhood abuse until they are in their thirties. Rarely do children report ongoing abuse. It's just too fearful and confusing for a child to handle. Out of eighty-six cases of incest reported to the Rape Response Center in Orlando, Florida, the average age of the person reporting was between thirty and forty-four. Many were married, had children, and were reporting being sexually abused as a child for the first time. It may be that the issue is brought out into the open to help someone else. In cases where the abuser is still active, adult survivors of abuse do for their children what they couldn't do for themselves and call for help.

There is also the possibility that the issue doesn't come up until the person is strong enough to cope with it. During the tumultuous and often erratic search for identity that is most peoples' journey through their twenties, the secret tends to sleep. Its emergence then might create too much chaos, and lacking a strong identity, the person would tend to go immediately into denial, burying the secret even deeper.

I have observed that people get unstuck when the discomfort of making a decision not to change their lives becomes too great. They finally take that long-delayed action because the chronically unhappy relationship, the dead-end job, the feelings of shame and guilt, and the lack of zest for life become too painful to continue. I have seen people in their sixties and seventies enter recovery; it's never too late to get the message and start the journey.

Suddenly the Memory Returns

When you finally feel safe enough, your secret steps quietly out of the shadows. The information is astonishing in its familiarity—an authentic and recognizable moment from your past. Sometimes people are surprised that up until that moment they had not remembered the significant event at all; others are equally astonished that they had not given it proper significance. What is most important, however, is not the specifics of the returned memory but the feelings around it that surface as well.

It wasn't until I went into a treatment center at the age of thirty-three that I felt safe enough to deal with my secrets. At a psychodrama exercise we were told to write a secret on a piece of paper, something we had never revealed to anyone. When I wrote, "My grandfather incested me," the words started to shake before my eyes. I realized it was my hands. I folded my secret in half and in half again and threw the piece of paper into the middle of a circle, full of dread and near panic over what I had written. One by one, members of the group drew from the pile of paper and read a secret aloud, then talked about it as if it were their own. When I heard someone else read those words, I was immediately flooded with tears. No one needed to wonder whose secret had been revealed. I cried and cried as the person who chose my secret described my life. He had also been a victim of incest, so the details he chose to tell my story came straight from his own most painful experience. He spoke of my secret in terms of loss—loss of childhood, loss of joy, of heart, of trust. He cried himself, for all my losses and the tragic impact the incest had on my life in terms of the shame I had to hide and the feelings of low value I had to live with.

As my flood of tears continued with the force of a waterfall dammed up for many years, people all around the circle kept discussing my secret. Hearing about it in the third person—removed from myself and reflected on by others—the events began to make a curious kind of sense to me. Before, I could never regard the incest logically because the information I had stored was all distorted. No matter how I tried to "figure it out," I ended up feeling bad. What struck me the most was that when people talked about the incest, their thinking was completely different from my own. They gave me a brand-new message that changed my life: that what my grandfather did was a terrible thing rather than that I was a terrible person. That message was what I couldn't get over, and the relief it brought is why the tears kept coming. Before I uncovered my secret, the only perception I had was my own, and it had been cruelly twisted by the shame I had assumed and by the defensive role playing I had done over the years in order to coexist with my secret. I was constantly, even obsessively, doing for others. I had to be good because I felt so bad about myself and my secret.

Having my secret reflected on by others instantly changed my perception. It was like getting the pieces of a difficult puzzle to finally fit together—suddenly they merge with ease and complete the picture. That picture was me without the shame, restored to my full value. The discovery was so delicious! As the hours and the days went by after my revelation, I kept feeling so wonderful. I remember thinking over and over, "I'm not alone any more. I'm not in pieces as I used to be." My discovery had a liberating effect on me. In the safety of the group, I felt what I could not feel as a child, and that experience changed me forever. For the first time I allowed myself to feel the pain and anger caused by my abuse that my childhood self couldn't handle and buried away. Feeling safe enough in the group to let those feelings surface rescued my spirit, the Real Me who had been in hiding for so long, and allowed her to come out into the light of the sun.

As my recovery progressed, I continued to experience the restoration of my core being in the form of enormous stores of good energy. I felt like the eager, dancing child I had once been who could enjoy life through every pore. All those years of struggling so hard to be good by doing good were over. Because I no longer felt tainted, the compulsion to be thought of as a good person had left me. *I* knew *I* was a good person, and that knowledge had always been what I needed.

The struggle to understand my grandfather's abuse was also over. There *was* no understanding it. No matter how hard I tried to figure it out, it couldn't be done. For years I kept trying to slay that same dragon again and again. Now that compulsion was gone, too. A kind of peace had been declared inside me, a truce from all the mental struggle, and in that peace the energy that used to go into protecting my secret went directly into what I needed for myself. I was open to life for the first time, ready to experience it to the full, and became so quickly caught up in the excitement that, in time, I rarely thought about my old obsessions at all.

However, I did keep talking about my secret, because every time I did, I found it helped someone. The more open about it I became, the better I felt. The negative energy of trying to always hide my secret slowly dissipated, as did all the feelings around the secret, to become just a small part of my core being. When the power of the secret was defused, everything attached to it—all my old fears and feelings of shame—lost its power, too. My energy now came from my spirit, pure and unadulterated.

There are many ways to jar loose a secret. In my case it involved powerful psychodrama, but it can also happen in a completely spontaneous way. In Marcel Proust's novel *Remembrance of Things Past,* the author recollects a sunny moment from his childhood in which the entire French country town of Combray and its environs had sprung vividly to mind when he dipped his little cake into a cup of tea. In Proust's description we see the shell-shaped madeleine, the color and smell of the tea, and feel and taste of the soaked buttery crumbs when swallowed. The combination of sensations reexperienced as an adult caused a flood of memory: "An exquisite pleasure had invaded my senses. . . . Suddenly the memory returns . . . the whole of Combray and its surroundings sprang into being, town and gardens alike, from my cup of tea."

Brain researchers now claim to have discovered how Proust's flood of memory is biochemically possible. Doctors Larry R. Squire and Stuart Zola-Morgan, of the University of California San Diego, studied the brain activity of a man whose hippocampus—an organ in the central brain—had been surgically removed to relieve epilepsy. The researchers found that the separate sensations that make up the memorable moment are first bound together in the hippocampus to become a heightened experience. The hippocampus then instructs the cells in the parts of the brain where the sensation originated to retain highly selective details of that memorable experience.

Memory becomes long-term with repetition. Each time the tea and madeleines are eaten, the hippocampus binds together the nerve messages into a memorable experience and then sends them back to be stored in the brain's complex filing system. After many recalls by the hippocampus, the memory becomes permanent. Then, experiencing a single sensation of the memory can recall the entire cluster of sensations and the accompanying rush of emotion—what Proust described as an invasion of exquisite pleasure.

When repressed material about a trauma is released in a flashback, we also become "flooded with memory." Like Proust's experience, the recollection is emotionally heightened but with fear rather than pleasure.

I find intriguing how consistently the details of the moment of a repressed memory are highly selective and always sensory, with a single sensation triggering a group of sensations that are experienced simultaneously in the flood. One could conjecture that the long-term memory of a trauma is stored in the same way the ecstasy of a childhood experience is stored, with a cup of tea and a madeleine the gateway to them all.

Flashbacks

When a person feels safe enough to deal with long-repressed information, up it comes. A flashback is difficult to describe to someone who hasn't experienced one. To say it appears like a visual memory, which can run in the mind like a scene on a movie screen, is to distance the experience. A flashback has no distance; it is the re-creation of the repressed trauma in all its immediacy and fright. The details are vivid and often appear enlarged. Their contents are undeniable.

Sometimes a flashback is experienced as a body memory, felt rather than seen. A patient of mine who had been penetrated as a child had always wondered why, whenever she heard of anyone being injured, she always felt a sympathetic pain in her vagina. At the release of her repressed memories, she began feeling these sharp pains as part of a flood of memory of the abuse, including where it happened and how. Medical doctors often talk about the high number of patients they diagnose as having psychosomatic illness. These patients complain of having pain, but their test results all run negative and nothing appears to be physically wrong. The doctors are right, for there is something spiritually, not physically, wrong. The symptoms are signals from the spirit through the body (because the mind won't listen) that something must be dealt with.

Delayed Understanding

Sometimes flashbacks are spontaneously triggered and seem to make no sense because a secret is so deeply buried. One woman in her fifties recalled her wedding night more than thirty years ago.

> My husband and I had fooled around to the limit during our engagement. It just about drove us crazy not to go all the way, but I was determined to be a virgin bride. We could both hardly wait to leave the ceremony and get to our hotel room, we were so turned on.
>
> But then the strangest thing happened. I never told anyone, even him, but as this guy whom I was so crazy for started coming toward the bed naked and I saw his genitals for the first time, I froze. The sight of them repelled me. I was in terror of them. It took weeks before that feeling went away. Now I know why the sight of my husband's approaching genitals filled me with terror—*I had seen that sight before.*

It would take two decades of therapy before she uncovered the source of her wedding night flashback: her father's repeated sexual abuse of her from age five to age seven.

In Its Own Time: Frank,
a Case History

When the brain begins to release its load of secrets, a person can rapidly begin to heal. I have become convinced that secrets don't emerge unless people feel safe enough to be able to feel their own powerlessness minus all the defenses that they have used to protect themselves for so long. People who have traumatic memories especially need to know that if they go back in time and dredge up something awful that they will be believed, comforted, and protected.

The mind is reluctant to unleash secrets without the element of safety. People can go through treatment time and again or through years of therapy or through decades of recovery programs, but if they never feel safe, they will never learn the truth about themselves. When the brain finally does let go of the floodgates of memory, however, the healing that takes place is truly and observably amazing. Once the secrets are allowed out in the open, the negative energy attached to secrets is defused and disappears like a puff of noxious air.

Frank is an example of a late bloomer who couldn't find an environment safe enough in which to unload his secret until he went into treatment at the age of sixty-one, after his eyesight began to fail him and he had persistent thoughts of suicide. Frank had felt stuck for a long time. He had sixteen years of abstinence from drinking and was a pillar of his local support group. "But in all my years of sobriety, I never got happy. I was able to stop drinkin' but I wasn't able to stop thinkin'," he says in his straightforward New England way. "Finally it got to the point where I didn't want to live anymore. When I started losing my eyesight, I asked my family doc to recommend a suicide doctor, and he made arrangements on the spot to get me into treatment.''

When I met Frank, he had been in treatment nine days and had made his first discovery. (A second, even more deeply buried secret had yet to make itself known.) Initially, he was one of those closed-down people whose early memories are few. Most of Frank's earliest recollections were of the family huddled around the living room radio worrying over the latest news from the fronts during World War II. His oldest brother never came back from the war. Another brother and two uncles were given a hero's parade down the main street of their small Massachusetts town.

Those really were the good old days, growing up in the years following World War II. People had jobs, money in their pockets; things were good. My father put a whole bottle of whiskey on the kitchen table. We ate meat and butter. These were all a status of wealth. Before I came to this hospital, I had always seen myself as having a happy, wonderful childhood, but now I know that was a big lie.

I grew up listening to the hunting and beer drinking stories of many older brothers and uncles. I remember feeling so bad when they described how animals were killed, but it was obvious I was the only one who felt that way. So I kept my mouth shut and believed I must be a daisy because this talk bothered me so much.

When I was eighteen, I volunteered to serve in the Korean War. Everybody I knew was there, and they were dying like flies in the first part of the war. I volunteered for Ranger training because I wanted to be tough. I was still worried about being a daisy and had found out that in the army you learned to bury your feelings, and that's just what I wanted to do. In training I saw guys break down, crying, "I can't make it. I can't go on." And they'd throw them right off the base like they were a piece of garbage. I'd think, "He left and I didn't. I'm really tough after all."

It was in the army that my drinking career began, on a cook's big jug of grain alcohol and grapefruit juice—the greatest elixir I have ever experienced. Once I met that cook, everything was bearable. I never wanted for a drink or went through a lot of pain in the army again.

I was sent to Korea as a radar repairman, not a soldier, but when the Chinese came south in a massive attack, I became involved in combat. Some of the kids in the Chinese army were fourteen or fifteen years old and even younger. They didn't have any medics or doctors. They just shot their wounded rather than take care of them. It was accepted as being normal for the Chinese, but it wasn't for me. I couldn't accept it. I saw a little kid get run over by an ammunition truck. "Keep moving," they said, and I thought to myself, "Nobody seems to have feelings over this, yet I do. What's wrong with me?"

I would wake up in a foxhole when the enemy would start shelling and think, "What the hell am I doing here?" We'd all run for the bunker, and the only thing in there were cases and cases of beer. Outside the bunker, the enemy would be screaming as they came up the side of the hill, and our commanding officer would yell, "Shoot, shoot! Don't even aim! Spray it!" We'd be pumping lead into them, and they'd be dropping like flies, running right over the dead ones, and it didn't bother anybody. No feelings. No feelings allowed.

I think part of my reason for volunteering for the army was to be able to handle this stuff, these feelings that weren't allowed in a man. But all I learned was I *couldn't* handle it. The feelings stayed. Images would haunt me, especially the young boy and the truck. I was haunted by the belief that there was something wrong with me because these images lingered. I'm aware now that because there's something *right* with me these things bothered me, but at the time I thought just the opposite.

After I was discharged, I met and married a nurse who tried to get me to go to an AA meeting. I insisted my drinking was under control—a couple of beers and that was it. When the kids came along, I kept that strict control of the booze, but as they got older, I found there were certain situations in which I just had to be drinking, like out in the woods when I took them camping. My canteen full of Southern Comfort was off limits to the kids.

Although I could control my drinking, I couldn't control my night terrors. I fought the war again and again in my sleep and would wake up exhausted from running all night in bed. My thrashing around kept my wife awake until finally we got twin beds. As time went by, the nights got worse and so did my drinking. I walked into an AA meeting sixteen and a half years ago next month and never took another drink. I found a power outside of myself in this group. That was good. But sobriety only worked while I was awake. My night terrors didn't go away, they got worse.

I went to get some help for what they were calling post-traumatic stress at the veteran's office on the main street of my hometown. A vet was sitting there listening quietly in a meeting with other vets and suddenly he spun around, took aim with a gun he had been concealing, and sprayed the back wall with holes. And we just went on talking! To this day, there are several holes in the back wall. Lots of men act violent rather than face this stuff. I just kept hurting.

I talked to the psychiatrist at the VA hospital about my nightmares about the war. He told me, "That was a long time ago. Let a sleeping dog lie." But it wouldn't lie. It was stuck in my mind. Just when I would fall into sleep and my guard was down, boom—I could see the dust after the truck went over that kid. But it was different, because now I felt for him what I couldn't let myself feel then.

I couldn't sleep with my wife any more because I kept waking her up with my constant trips to the bathroom or the kitchen for relief. We finally had to sleep in separate bedrooms. It was the first in a series of losses that sent me here. Next, my health started to break down, one thing after another—a stroke, diabetes, and then my eyes—but no one ever put all these things together and said, "Frank, what's the problem?" And even if they had, I couldn't have told them. It got to the point where I just didn't want to live any more. I went to my family doctor and asked him if he could recommend me to one of those suicide doctors. I wanted to go out quietly and with as little fuss as possible. He got together with my wife, and they put me in here.

By the end of the first week of treatment, as I started getting those feelings around my war experience expressed in group, I was sleeping like a baby, the first good sleep of my life. I got a lot of that negative energy discharged, but the real secret, the one doing the most damage, was still buried. Then one day in group this memory just flashed before my eyes:

I was eight or nine and standing in my uncle's driveway. He raised Irish hunting dogs, the kind with short curly hair, bred to point and heel when given the command. When they didn't obey, my uncle destroyed them. I saw the scene in my mind as clearly as if I were really standing there in the driveway today instead of fifty years ago. And I watched my uncle kill a dog, just shot him like it was nothing—this beautiful dog who was really good as far as I was concerned—and I told myself, it doesn't matter. I also knew that I had seen this cruel sight many times before, as if I made a point of watching, as if somehow watching would help make me a man.

Discovery

I'll never forget the day I met Frank, shortly after the discovery of his most deeply buried secret. He was in a group session sitting tall in his chair, like a military man even in his lounging clothes, with a little stuffed animal on his knee. When people asked him about his spotted dog, he would reply, "This is Ralph. He doesn't hunt."

By the end of treatment, Frank had worked through the shame over his sensitivity to a cruel environment. Although at first he was only able to feel strongly for animals, gradually he was able to feel for the little boy inside of him whose gentleness was not valued. Frank no longer runs in bed at night. He has found a new lightness of being. He looks back on his path through life and is in awe of the strength of his convictions that seemed to self-germinate in a hostile environment and the way those convictions persisted even though they were suppressed for decades.

Six months after treatment, Frank is out enjoying life and, after another setback with his heart, zealous about living the no-fat way. Now, instead of the burden he had felt life was, his greatest challenge is to enjoy the changing seasons. He, his wife, daughter, and grandchild had taken a drive up to Vermont when the leaves were changing. "Each tree was a flower," he told me excitedly. "I experience life more intensely now. I'm more aware. I can't see any better but what I do see, I see more deeply. I can enjoy life more because I don't do those things that drive me crazy. I have no more trouble sleeping, and so each night I'm out like a baby and refreshed each morning. I don't take credit for it, but I think I influenced my daughter to turn her life around. She's back in college. All in all, I feel my life is about ten thousand percent better."

The Time Comes When It Comes

People like Frank take a long time uncovering their secrets because they are so concerned they are not going to be accepted. Out of a need for the acceptance of his family and his culture, Frank buried his real self and all the feelings surrounding the abuse of animals that bothered him so much. In pushing down his secret, Frank lost his sense of identity. He became disconnected from his spirit. He stayed that way for a long time until he found an environment where his fears melted away.

Once you are in a safe place where you receive love and caring, your real identity starts to blossom, and all this stuff, the repressed information and all its disturbing negative energy, is going to emerge. It will come up because your spirit wants to be reconnected to you, but it has been blocked by fear and your repressed feelings. In expressing those feelings in a safe place, you will set your spirit free.

ACTIVITIES
Days 12-18

Day 12: Early Sexual Messages

1. What was the first fear you can remember ever having about sex?

2. Describe a sexual message you received from your parents and how it manifests itself in your current sexual behavior or lack of sexual activity.

Day 13: Early Sexual Messages—A Guided Imagery

An early sexual message may be visual, or it may be a feeling. This exercise will help put these messages in focus so they can be identified. Lie or sit comfortably and close your eyes. Inhale slowly and deeply. Exhale completely. Repeat four times. If you are feeling particularly stressed, do the progressive relaxation exercise from Day Six (page 46). Imagine yourself when you were young, living at home, at a family gathering, or in your neighborhood. Notice people coming into the scene and approaching you. What do you see, hear, feel? What are the adults around you doing? Are they acting affectionately or otherwise? What early sexual messages, spoken or unspoken, are you receiving? What major message keeps coming back to you about sex? What are you seeing or hearing sexually? What are you experiencing at this moment? If the message is in the form of a feeling, where in your body do you feel it?

Write down one dominant experience from the imagery. List the early sexual message you received and the resulting feelings you experienced. Here is an example: A woman remembered exploring her genitals after a bath and being surprised by her mother, after which she remembered nothing. The feelings she experienced were fear and shame.

Write in your journal how these early sexual messages have affected your life. Examples might be people pleasing, stomach pains, sexual numbness, promiscuity, seductiveness, compulsive masturbation, or fear of intimacy.

Then write down how your life would change if you were to reject these early sexual messages. What have you learned about yourself from exploring these messages?

Day 14: Hidden Anger

We hide our anger because we are conditioned to believe it is undesirable at best and sinful or destructive at worst. Women, especially, are taught to avoid getting angry, which, of course, is not possible. Being unaware of your anger does not mean you are not angry. In fact, it is the anger you are unaware of that can do the most damage to you and your relationships. When you do finally express your repressed negative feelings, they won't be in the form of irritation, annoyance, or "getting mad," but full-blown rage that takes over your whole being.

Discharging anger by going from zero to rage is an inappropriate response that only does more harm. We need to learn to recognize the feelings when they are still manageable, acknowledge them as legitimately ours, and act on those feelings in some appropriate way. Undischarged, anger gets refueled as resentment, the number one characteristic of the addictive person. We cannot afford the luxury of resentment.

Everybody has ways of signaling the presence of angry feelings. Look for your ways. Ask others who care about you to help you because they may be able to observe your irritation before you become aware of it. Some common bodily signals are clamming up;

blushing; shallow breathing; drumming fingers; foot tapping; shaking or twisting; laughing when nothing amusing is happening; patting or stroking the back of the head; clenching jaws or fist; tucking a thumb inside of a fist; yawning or getting drowsy; sudden refusal to make eye contact; giving an apology when none is asked for; headaches; pains in the neck, stomach, or back; and a rise or a fall in voice pitch.

Other forms of expression may be more subtle or creative, like suddenly saying "I think I'll paint the house today." Discharging anger that way may result in getting tasks done, but it does nothing to help the unexpressed feelings.

We often mask our anger to such an extent that we lose the ability to recognize the fact that we are angry until it has exploded into rage. The following checklist has been designed to assist you in identifying ways you may be hiding your anger from yourself as well as others.

Put a check next to the following statements with which you identify:

_____ 1. Procrastination in the completion of imposed tasks.

_____ 2. Perpetual or habitual lateness.

_____ 3. A liking for sadistic or ironic humor.

_____ 4. Sarcasm, cynicism, or flippancy in conversation.

_____ 5. Overpoliteness, constant cheerfulness, or an attitude of "grin and bear it."

_____ 6. Frequent sighing.

_____ 7. Smiling when hurting.

_____ 8. Frequent disturbing or frightening dreams.

_____ 9. An overcontrolled, monotone speaking voice.

_____10. Difficulty in getting to sleep or sleeping through the night.

_____11. Boredom, apathy, or a loss of interest in things you are usually excited about.

_____12. Slowing down of movements.

_____13. Getting tired more easily than usual.

_____14. Excessive irritability over trifles.

_____15. Getting drowsy at inappropriate times.

_____16. Sleeping more than usual—maybe twelve to fourteen hours a day.

_____17. Waking up tired rather than rested and refreshed.

_____18. Clenched jaws, especially when sleeping.

_____19. Facial tics, spasmodic foot movements, habitual fist clenching, and similar repeated physical acts done unintentionally.

_____20. Grinding of the teeth, especially when sleeping.

_____21. Chronically stiff or sore neck or shoulder muscles.

_____22. Chronic depression—extended periods of feeling down for no reason.

_____23. Stomach ulcers.

Write in your journal about the characteristics of hidden anger you identify with the strongest. Describe any new ways you have just discovered that you use to express your hidden anger. What are additional ways you may hide your anger that are not on the list?

Passive–aggressive behavior is another manifestation of repressed anger; it is the deepest hidden anger of all. A pattern of *not* saying or doing something, which results in problems for others—not conveying a message or not mailing an important letter—is a form of hidden or passive–aggressive anger you will be able to find if you can be totally honest with yourself.

Here is an example of passive–aggressive anger in action in a relationship: A husband and wife occupy a very small apartment. She goes to bed earlier than he does and is kept up by the noise of the television and his "puttering around." However, she is too insecure to complain. Instead, she comes back to bed noisily after going to the bathroom at 6 A.M., vigorously punching her pillow and "thrashing around," as he describes it, to get comfortable. He doesn't complain either. Both are only vaguely aware of how much their sleep pattern is being disturbed and how angry they are at each other for not being able to pick up on their subtle clues.

Remember this: Regardless of the way anger is expressed or not expressed, it emanates from loss. The next time you feel angry, instead of asking yourself why you're feeling angry, ask yourself what you've lost. Your answer may come to you readily and your feelings turn into an expression of that loss.

Day 15: Dream Themes

One person I know has a recurring dream of packing his suitcase to go somewhere. He is frantically, hopelessly late, looking for clothes and shoes, trying to read an incomprehensible airline ticket, trying to dial a phone and unable to read the strangely coded numbers. Another person, a long-time people pleaser, frequently dreams of serving dinner to a huge crowd of people, with more arriving to take the place of those who have finished, as she scurries around the kitchen, washing dishes, cutting up onions, pouring coffee, and sick with the knowledge that she can't possibly feed them all.

When these people I know so well tell me their dreams, I see how accurately they portray themselves. The frantic traveler has been stuck for a long time, his life constantly put on hold to follow someone else's agenda—first that of spouse and children and now that of aging parents. The frantic cook is a people pleaser and a doer big time. It doesn't help her situation that she's also a very good cook. However, nobody gets to appreciate the dinners she serves in her dreams, and they leave her exhausted by morning.

Some dreams leave more than an emotional impact. Each time they recur, they cause the dreamer to wake in fear, shot through with adrenaline, and to feel depressed the next day. The dreams have a predictable pattern. One patient repeatedly dreamed of climbing to the top of a ladder then experiencing a sudden terrifying fall. Another found herself in her dreams being in a familiar place that became frighteningly unfamiliar or in a tight place where there wasn't enough air to breathe.

Write in your journal about any themes you may find in your dream life, disturbing or otherwise. Recording these themes is the first step to discovering the secret they may contain. Concentrate on their emotional impact. What feelings do they bring up as you write them down?

Day 16: Behind the Mask—Dysfunctional Family Roles

When we are out of control we play roles, old familiar roles that emanate from the ones we played in our families long before we created protective disguises for our adult selves to wear in public. These childhood roles were created in order to survive in dysfunctional families, and although not every dysfunctional family has a member for every role, every person in the family must take on at least one role in order to perpetuate the dysfunction.

I define a dysfunctional family as one in which expression of a person's core being is not allowed. We take on roles as a way to keep our spirits alive. The problem is, as adults, when we are out of control, we fall back into these roles. Being out of control is a hard place to be, and these old familiar disguises give us a familiar base of security, a way to be, but in the process we give up our identity, choices, and our feelings. We become like children again.

The following roles—the hero, the scapegoat, the lost child, and the mascot—are stereotypical roles frequently played in dysfunctional families. As you read the descriptions, you may identify with one or more of the roles. You may also be able to recognize roles played by other family members. The problem with roles we learn to play at home is that we get stuck playing them out in the world as well. We seem to unwittingly absorb the old family patterns and take them into the world where we transfer them to all the relationships we have. If you take a close look at the following roles that are commonly developed in dysfunctional families, you may be able to see how you have taken on some of these patterns into your adult life. Be grateful for this discovery, for now the pattern can be broken.

FOOD FOR LOVE

The Hero

The hero fulfills a family's need for a good self-image by being successful. A hero gives the family cause to feel proud by superachieving in school, sports, or business or with a special talent. Heroes are usually the ones who are the most aware of what's really happening in the family and assume responsibility for making things better. For that reason, there are a lot of firstborn heroes, who, by nature of being mommy's little helper, assume the caretaker role. If one or both parents are irresponsible, the hero takes care of them, too.

Heroes work very hard for approval and are often successful in other people's eyes. Heroes get Ph.D.'s in impression management. Because they assume too much responsibility, however, they are unable to really enjoy their success. If they become addicted, it is more often to food or work than alcohol or drugs. They are also more likely to develop eating disorders. On the down side, heroes are rigid, manipulative, and controlling. They can never be wrong.

On the outside, heroes appear to be the soul of competence. On the inside, heroes feel progressively inadequate, confused, and angry at all the responsibility they assume to overcompensate for irresponsible family members. They are lonely and empty because they feel there is no one they can share their burdens with.

In recovery, heroes learn to accept failure and become responsible for themselves first and then others on a practical, as-needed basis. They become more balanced in the time they spend at work and at play and do not identify themselves by what they accomplish. They redefine success to include happiness. Heroes excel at being executives. (One study of sixty-five chief executive officers revealed that 75 percent were firstborn.) In recovery, they learn to use their high energy to serve themselves rather than maintain the family image.

QUESTIONS: Is there a member of your family who plays the hero role? If not, can you speculate why? If so, when was the role assumed and why? If you play the hero, how did reading this make you feel? How has playing the hero hindered you in your life outside the family? How has it helped you? What qualities have you developed playing the hero that you can put to good use serving yourself?

The Scapegoat

In dysfunctional families, there is room for only one hero. The scapegoat, like the child born after the first-son-and-heir, must break new ground to find an identity. Scapegoats show more cynicism about the way the family functions and do not buy into the family need for a positive identity. Scapegoats are not willing to put all that effort into what they see as an unfair game in which no one is valued for who they really are. At the first opportunity, they may distance themselves from the family, emotionally and geographically, to seek new associations.

The scapegoat gives the family distraction, taking the focus of blame off other members. As they are often absent from the home, they become a convenient suspect for anything bad that happens. Although they are openly treated with contempt by family members, scapegoats are secretly highly valued, for they can be blamed for all the dysfunction, and the other family members don't have to examine their own behavior or change.

Some scapegoats do not escape from the clutches

of the family. Instead, they get caught up in playing the destructive side of their role because they find it is the only way they can get the attention they need. They get pregnant, become runaways, use drugs, make trouble in school, or commit crimes as a way of competing with the family hero for attention and recognition.

On the outside, scapegoats are rebellious, hostile, angry, and defiant. Or they are free spirits who don't care what you think. On the inside, they are hurt and full of guilt. When they carry their role out into the world, they get into so much trouble that they tend to retreat into self-preoccupation and solitary activity. They become defensive and paranoid as a result of all the times they have been unfairly accused.

In recovery, scapegoats are nonconformists who march to that different drummer. They are courageous, have high moral standards, and are able to accept reality without illusion. They no longer buy into guilt. They accept responsibility for themselves and place a high value on their peers. They make good counselors. They have great senses of humor.

QUESTIONS: Does anyone in your family play the scapegoat role? If not, speculate on why not. If so, when was it assumed and why? If you play the scapegoat, how did reading this make you feel? How has playing the scapegoat hindered you in your life outside the family? How has it helped you? What qualities have you developed playing the scapegoat that you can put to good use serving yourself?

The Lost Child

Relief is the lost child's gift to the family—that at least one person isn't causing trouble. They are the quiet children the other members don't pay much attention to in either a positive or a negative way. Lost children have learned to refrain from trying to bond with members of the family and keep to themselves. Like heroes, they are likely to have eating disorders. They are commonly found in large families, but they can also be found in small families where undue attention is focused on others, as in a family where one child has a disability or is precocious.

On the outside, the lost child appears quiet, aloof, superindependent, and mildly contented. On the inside, the lost child feels lonely, hurt, angry, and inadequate. However, these feelings are completely covered up by the lost child's seeming preference for going it alone.

Lost children grow up with a low-energy approach to life. They have problems with isolation and an insecure sexual identity and may remain single seemingly by choice. They sometimes die at an early age.

In recovery, lost children bloom: They have already developed so many creative and imaginative ways to entertain themselves, they are a joy in a group. Now they begin to express their talents to the rest of the world. Because they are independent self-starters, they make good entrepreneurs. They learn to value people.

QUESTIONS: Does anyone in your family play the role of the lost child? If not, can you speculate why not? If so, which member plays this role? When was it assumed and why? If you are a lost child, how did reading this make you feel? How has playing the lost child hindered you in your life outside the family? How has it helped you? What qualities have you developed playing the role that you can put to good use serving yourself?

FOOD FOR LOVE

The Mascot

It seems the mascot is born cute and with a sense of fun. From early on, these qualities are encouraged by a dysfunctional family desperate for a little comic relief. As adults, mascots are the ones in their group family picture clowning around. Younger children especially are often compelled to play the mascot way beyond the time when it is appropriate for them to be so superadorable.

Mascots develop a thousand ways to attract your attention. They are expected to provide entertainment, but no one takes mascots seriously when they are in distress. In fact, expressing their bad feelings will provoke another round of laughter. As a result, mascots stay superficial and childlike because mature behavior has been actively discouraged.

On the outside, the mascot appears to be charming, lovable if fragile, full of energy, and magnetically attractive. On the inside, mascots are angry, lonely, confused, and fearful of rejection. They are furious over not being taken seriously.

Like heroes, mascots are high-energy people. They may even be hyperactive. They grow up charming and full of fun, but they also may have learning disabilities, a short attention span, and an inability to handle stress. Their clowning becomes compulsive, perpetuating the belief that they are immature. They often marry heroes for care and protection.

In recovery, mascots retain their wonderful, wacky senses of humor that provide so much enjoyment, but they grow up. They are still fun to be with, but they learn to take care of themselves and find that the need to entertain others is optional. Mascots learn to express their serious sides in a way that others can absorb, and their new balanced approach to life makes them deep and meaningful. The ability to laugh is one of God's greatest gifts. Mascots are fortunate to have received that gift early in life instead of having to nurture it along the way the hero, scapegoat, and lost child often must in recovery.

QUESTIONS: Does anyone in your family play this role? If not, can you speculate why not? If so, which member plays this role? When was it assumed and why? If you are a mascot, how did reading this make you feel? How has playing the mascot hindered you in your life outside the family? How has it helped you? What qualities have you developed playing the role that you can put to good use serving yourself?

The dysfunctional family cannot perpetuate the status quo unless all members play their roles compulsively and in character, and no one breaks through the wall of delusion. Should a single member step outside the system and insist on the right to form an identity, the family will go into crisis. Each member is guaranteed to react with a great deal of defensiveness.

If you are preparing to break out of your role, take a moment to imagine the reactions of each family member and describe what each has to lose when you give up playing your dysfunctional role. By breaking out, what have you got to win?

If you have found patterns in the role you played in your dysfunctional family that you have transferred to your life outside the family, imagine how you could deal with problems and relationships without the handicap of your dysfunctional family role.

Survivors of dysfunctional families are the strongest people I know, because they grew up learning skills that allowed them to survive within their family. Recovery is drawing on those strengths to work *for* you, not against you, and not just to survive and perpetuate the family dysfunction, but to live a meaningful life with meaningful relationships.

Day 17: What's Your Theme Song?

I have learned that music is one of the best ways to cut through people's defenses and get to their emotions. This is particularly true in men. In fact, it seems one of the few ways men will allow themselves to express feelings is by singing lyrics. Music may be universal, but theme songs are as individualistic as a scent. Like a favorite perfume, a person's theme song somehow underscores the essence of who they are.

Does a theme song come to mind? If not, I want you to take some time out to find your theme song. It may be connected with a happy memory, or it may be about something you really care about, a cause, or a part of the country. It may be one of those songs that makes you cry for no reason or makes you want to get up and dance. Once you've settled on a theme song, dance to it as part of your daily exercise. Learn all the verses and sing it in the shower. Why did you choose this song? Draw a picture of your theme song.

Day 18: The House of Joy

The following is a poem written by a patient at "Your Life Matters." If you find comfort or meaning in it, you may want to copy it down in your journal.

I am leaving the House of Pain
Where intimacy is forbidden

88

Discovery

A house where no one knows my name
And secrets must be hidden.
I am moving into the House of Joy
Where hurtfulness is forbidden
And my Spirit is fully employed
To Heal what has been hidden.

III

The Special Problems
of Sexual Abuse

An Aching in My Heart:
Janet's Story

I grew up in the Red Hook section of Brooklyn, where, as everywhere, kids found lots of opportunity to explore their natural sexual curiosity. The little boys and girls in my neighborhood would occasionally go into the bushes and play a game called "you show me yours and I'll show you mine." It felt dangerous as a kid. As a therapist, I have heard the game described so many times it makes me wonder whether this secret form of "show but don't tell" is a universal childhood ritual.

When I was five, a bunch of us kids were caught in the bushes playing the show-me game by a little boy's mom. My heart can still race when I recall the shock of that awful moment of discovery, and I can still feel the shame that followed when the news reached my mother, to say nothing of the spanking I got at home.

However, the source of that first fearful imprint about sex, which was to have such a powerful impact on the rest of my life, was not about getting caught in the bushes. It came from my mother's warning about sex that followed. With urgency in her voice, she explained to me what a virgin was and how every girl had what was called a cherry. "Boys are always going to be after you for it," she warned me, "and it's what most men really want." I had to be always on my guard, for a boy could be talking to me about anything but what was really on his mind was sex. I took this early negative message into adulthood and was constantly fearful around men. A need for protection took precedence over a desire for intimacy.

The great irony of my childhood is that when I was exploring my sexuality in what I now regard as a perfectly healthy and appropriate way, I was caught in the act, punished, and publicly humiliated, but the sexual acts I was a party to, which *should* have been made public and were toxically harmful to my well-being, remained a secret, and the offender, my grandfather, went to his grave unpunished and unhumiliated. Having to keep my grandfather's secret was a special problem, as is often the case with sexual abuse. When a parent hits a child, there is no doubt in most children's minds that such an act is wrong. When a child is sexually abused, however, that sense of right and wrong is obscured. Only the need for secrecy is clear.

Before I began attending school, my mother returned to work. My grandmother also had a job, so my grandfather would take care of me. We had a ritual. First we'd hit the bars, where he had been taking me since I was a curly-haired little kid who was only too happy to perform a song and dance act on top of the table for the customers. My grandfather was your typical charming Irish drunk, the entertaining type everybody in a bar is glad to see. In fact, he was so charming, he hardly worked a day in his life.

The bars were exciting places. In each one, I'd perform my little Shirley Temple number, urged on by my grandfather, and give the money I got from the customers for my performance to my grandfather. He would then use the money to get drunk. As we made the rounds, my grandfather would drink at each bar, becoming more and more jovial. It was all so fun. Then we'd go home.

Alone in the house, he'd say to me, "Let's take a nap." I dreaded those naps. I knew his fondling had to be wrong because he kept reminding me not to tell anyone. I hated what he did to me, but at the same time—and this is what is so hard for me to understand—I adored him. I really loved him and bonded with him more than anyone else in my family. Everyone wanted his love, and at times he felt more important to me than my own father. In spite of his abuse of me, I *wanted to be like him*. Everyone liked him.

My grandfather was a very shrewd man; he seduced me into loving him deeply. He gave me anything I wanted and spoiled me with attention. He bought me every imaginable kind of stuffed animal. Although he had eighteen grandchildren, he always told me I was his favorite—the smartest, the cutest, the most fun to be with. When he talked to me about "our little secret," I felt special, and it was exciting to get away with something that nobody else knew about. I guess I decided it was all right to have secrets with people you loved.

There was another reason I kept his secret. When

I was just learning to talk, I became a menace to my parents because I would tell the neighbors everything. Once I announced to them with glee that my mom and dad were fighting. "You should see my mother yelling!" I told them. That day I got a strong message from my parents that I shouldn't tell anybody our business. I had developed a reputation as a "gabby gal," and I was sternly lectured about not revealing something that had happened at home to the outside world. That admonition added to the weight of the burden I carried about keeping quiet about what my grandfather did to me.

Nevertheless, the secret haunted me. I knew what he did was wrong, but I had no way of knowing how wrong or what the norms were. Even if I had been able to make a judgment, I was just a little kid! I couldn't have been able to make sense of the situation, for my sexual perception had already been distorted by my mother's fearful messages. When I had been caught in the bushes playing my childish game, I was punished, but here was my grandfather doing something that had to be wrong and he would never be punished. I thought that even if I told people, I wouldn't be believed—I was just a little kid and my grandfather was held in high esteem by so many people. I just couldn't make sense of it: Why were my actions in the bushes wrong while my grandfather's little games were unpunishable?

There was yet another twist to my childhood sexual development. I had completely repressed the memory until I began writing this chapter, but then it popped almost instantaneously into my mind as a clear and vivid picture of the Brooklyn street I lived on. We had moved to another section of Brooklyn called Park Slope. Like every other kid in the neighborhood, I was always looking for ways to earn a little money, and one of the few opportunities available was going to the store for the neighbors. At that time, every block in Park Slope was like a little extended family. Most of the people on my street were related to me in one way or another. Nobody thought anything of sending their children to the grocery store, even ones as young as six or seven like myself. I would run their errands and the neighbors would pay me with spare change; I also returned their empty soda bottles and got to keep the deposit money.

There was a very obese man who always sat outside a local dentist's office at the end of my block—the man I'd forgotten about all these years. He used to pay me much more than the others for going to the store, as much as twenty-five and even fifty cents. He would send me to buy him cigarettes, and when I'd come back with them, he would expose himself. I never said anything to him; I didn't even react. It was very clear in my mind that what this neighbor was doing was wrong; I had no feelings of love for him to confuse me as in the situation with my grandfather. Nevertheless, every time the man exposed himself, he made *me* feel dirty—as if I had done something wrong.

His indecent act didn't bother me as much as the fact that I pretended nothing happened. I kept going to the store for him because I wanted the money, all the while ashamed of this terrible thing I was doing for a little extra change. When it came to my own behavior, I seemed to have an overactive conscience, a sense of overresponsibility, that focused not on the behavior of the offender but on the feeling that there was something very wrong with me. Instead of seeing this neighbor as a dirty old man, I saw myself as a dirty little kid. I had never received the message that sexual curiosity and confusion were a normal response. I had no conception of normal. All I knew was anything sexual left me feeling tainted and unacceptable.

Eventually one of the other children in the neighborhood reported the exposer to the police. I could have done the same, and maybe if I hadn't had the experience with my grandfather, I would have said something, but I had already been put in a moral dilemma of *not telling*. Even when it was clear to me that someone was doing something wrong, I couldn't act. Reflecting back, I know that I internalized any sexual abuse, and it felt like my fault.

Another special problem of sexual abuse is it makes a second disconnection, not only from the spirit but also from the spiritual. I sought refuge in church for my guilty feelings, but I was rarely comforted. I loved the ritual of lighting candles for Saint Theresa. There was a statue of her in the church I was baptized in, and she was a favorite of the women in my family because she was the saint you turned to for help in little things. People left her roses. Mostly I felt inferior and ashamed in church because of the sexual abuse and never prayed or felt I really belonged there. Because I wore a mantle of shame when I went to mass, I was unable to make a connection with the spiritual there. My loss of faith—that I lived in a world where such things were done to a child and there was no justice—robbed me of my child's right to innocence and kept me isolated from any possibility of a spiritual connection. My shame would not allow it.

When I look into the eyes of myself as a child in family photographs, they seem to know too much. They seem to be far older than the rest of my face, and my brow is not smooth and untroubled the way a child's brow is supposed to be. When I look at that little worried face, I know now that I never felt like a child. How could I? My innocence had been ripped away. I was invaded by a knowledge of sexuality that was supposed to be revealed to me far off in a distant future of adulthood, when I was prepared to deal with it.

Because I did not feel like a child, I could not act like a child. After hearing my mother's warning about men and their sexuality (a far cry from the usual lecture about the birds and the bees, which would have been appropriate for my age), I couldn't say, "But I'm just a little kid. Protect me!" Instead I thought I had to protect her. In retrospect, I see how much damage I perceived would be done by telling my mother something I knew she would think was awful. It seemed to me that my mother's family was her whole world. If I told her my secret, I would ruin her life. I kept my silence.

All through my childhood, I swallowed the secret every time it rose within me and tried very hard to bury it deep enough where it wouldn't bother anyone, but it bothered me. In the years of continued silence that followed, my secret became wordless, reduced to an aching in my heart that would not leave me, a feeling that I sometimes still experience today—a grieving for the loss of a little kid's world. I knew too much too soon, and that made all the difference.

I managed to suppress the entire issue of sexuality until I started developing. I was an early bloomer; at the age of twelve I was the first girl in my class to wear a bra, and soon my expanding chest was a favorite topic of conversation among the boys. As a child, I was seductive. I craved attention and wanted to be cute, to be all sorts of exciting things to men. As a twelve-year-old who could suddenly pass for sixteen or seventeen, I resumed the familiar seduction path

I had begun on the bartops with my grandfather. There were plenty of role models to emulate and one of mine was Marilyn Monroe. I became a sweater girl, and I flaunted it. Sexuality was a game to play as long as I didn't have sex or do anything "dirty."

Because I had always taken on a lot of responsibility at home, I had more liberties than the normal twelve-year-old. I was precocious in school and in my social life. All the girls I ran with were four and five years older than I. I loved sports, especially skating, and it was at the local rink that I discovered sailors. After skating, my friends and I would head for an ice cream parlor next to a bar where sailors frequented, and they would come over from the bar and sit with us. As my boobs continued to grow, I got more and more of their undivided attention.

I started dating a sailor who was twenty-six. I'm sure he had no idea I was only twelve. My first boyfriend would bring me to the bars, and I started drinking. I loved alcohol immediately—loved the way it turned the world into a foggy fantasy. Drinking also gave me a lot of relief from the bad feelings I had been swallowing down for so long. I took to bars like a duck to water. Ever since my Shirley Temple days when I danced on bartops all over the neighborhood to earn money for my grandfather's drinks, bars had held nothing but exciting memories for me. As usual, my parents didn't have a clue. They thought I was just going skating. My boyfriend and I kissed and fooled around a lot, but we never had sex. I had a deep fear of penetration.

At home, my changing body did not go unnoticed. My grandfather had always made comments about my body that made me feel ashamed and uncomfortable, and these new developments elicited even more remarks. My father, on the other hand, was very respectful. He talked gleefully about how attractive I was, what a brilliant mind I had, and how unique I was—able to do anything I wanted. Instead of becoming upset at my grandfather, I transferred the intensity of my feelings to my father, whose actions were never inappropriate. For some unexplainable reason, I became petrified about my father's comments about my body and started distancing myself from him. I created all sorts of reasons to hate him. I couldn't stand the way he talked or the way he ate, not even potatoes, and I developed a strong aversion to his body. Until my adolescence, my feelings for my father were pure and uncomplicated. Puberty changed that.

My father worked nights and woke up at four o'clock in the afternoon each day. Sometimes he would leave me a note asking me to wake him, as he had a hard time getting up. My father slept in the nude, and sometimes the blanket wasn't completely over him. I was so repulsed by the sight of his body because of my grandfather that it actually sickened me. Usually I would try to get my brother to wake him. To this day, I can't stand to wake anybody up, and I don't like to look at men's naked bodies the fascinated way men like to look at women's bodies in sexy magazines.

Now I see that part of my intense feelings toward my father had to do with fury at him for not protecting me. I would look at him absorbed in his book at the kitchen table and fling silent but furious accusations at him: You don't have a clue as to what I'm about or what's going on in your own house. How come you don't protect me? How come you don't care? How come you don't make sure that I am home on time? You keep inviting Grandpa to go to the race track with you all the time—how come you can't see what he has done to me? How could you keep wanting to spend time with him?

Instead of saying anything, I left clues. For instance, I made sure I was never alone with my grandfather. If he ever came upon me when I was alone, I found an immediate excuse to leave his presence. My father's days off were Tuesday and Wednesday, and he and my grandfather often went to the race track then. Whenever my grandfather came to the house, I would leave. I was sure that even if my father was too naive to pick up on my behavior, my grandfather knew why I cleared out so fast. I could see by the look on his face that he knew.

I wouldn't even stay alone in a room with him and my grandmother because I doubted she could protect me. I thought my grandmother might know my secret. She was a very big woman, sweet but not very bright. She was like a child and passively let things happen. She felt so powerless to stop "something that men did" that she said nothing, just like me. Nevertheless, a tone in her voice when she would say "Where are you going?" or a look on her face or a kind of energy in her embrace told me that she knew.

I couldn't turn to anyone in my family for help and felt very alone. In my isolation, the only voice I heard was my own internal shaming: How could I still love my grandfather and want his attention more than I wanted my own father's? How could I continue to love him in spite of the things he had done? I was very comfortable around my "Poppa" as long as the whole family was there. I cherished the times when we were all together with him and I felt safe. He was brilliant without any real education, a patented inventor with a quick sense of humor who loved to tease. I found his love of bantering very attractive. His presence enlivened every gathering.

In my silent universe, my secret knowledge could be shared with no one. I saw myself as having no choice. Over the years, it had become an unspoken code of honor, a vow of integrity to myself, that I bear it alone.

Then, shortly after I had started drinking, my grandfather died. I drank at the funeral. I took his death very hard, and one of the hardest moments at the wake came when my mother said, "The bastard should have died years ago." I was shocked to hear her say that about someone who had just died and her father, no less. How dare she! I thought. Frequently I did not understand my mother's anger. She had a way of lashing out at my grandfather that upset me, and the way she treated her youngest brother, Eddie, who was one of the greatest guys in the family, had me mystified.

My drinking went out of control. I had regular blackouts. It was amazing that I managed to hold on to my virginity. By the time I was thirteen I was engaged to be married, diamond ring and all. By the age of seventeen, I had been engaged ten times and never had sex, because I was so petrified of the thought of being penetrated. I had managed to hold on by staying away from boys in the neighborhood. Getting involved with boys in the neighborhood and going through the usual dating rituals was too dangerous. It had been my observation that after two or three dates the pressure was on to have sex. Because I wouldn't give in to sex, it seemed as if I didn't have a lot of dates beyond the third one.

Sailors, on the other hand, would come and go, and there wasn't anything serious about them. They weren't so persistent about having sex like the macho boys in the neighborhood. I was able to keep sailors dangling and then when the pressure got too much, I would move on. A couple of the guys I knew talked about having platonic relationships. I used to wonder what they meant, for in my world there were no options. To have sex or not to have sex was the one and only quest. Any relationship with a man had to eventually involve penetration, and I wasn't prepared to deal with that.

I used my bustline as a distraction. Emphasized with sweaters, it was a focus of men's attraction wherever I went. Although I was detached from any feelings of pleasure in my body, at least I didn't have a fear attached to my breasts. However, it was hard keeping men focused on one part of me without involving their interest in the other. Although it felt good to be sexually attractive, it was only to lure them into a relationship, not to have sex.

In order to keep the upper hand, I had to be devious. The game was to be seductive, and then, when a guy really started coming on to me, I would get pleasure out of being able to say no. I enjoyed leaving them panting. I enjoyed the fact that they wanted me and I wasn't going to give in, and it never bothered me a bit that I had led them on. It was almost as if I were punishing them. In the meantime, I complained all the time that sex was all men wanted, my mother's childhood litany. During this crazy time of sexual acting out without having sex, there was no sensual enjoyment in any of it. I was detached from my body and had numbed any sexual desire with food or alcohol.

When I was seventeen I ran away from home on Easter Sunday, a symbolic choice. Every year until my grandfather died, I alone out of eighteen grandchildren had received an Easter basket and pile of stuffed animals from my grandfather, and every year I used to wonder, Doesn't this give any of you a clue? Can't you figure out what's going on?

I kept my secret until I was thirty-three years old. I stuffed it down with food until I weighed 350 pounds. I wore disguises, posing as a chronic doer to hide my shame. I drank when food was not enough to give me relief. I got involved with men who I thought I could love, but I never let any of them really touch me. Because of my grandfather's abuse and my mother's negative messages I kept all men at an emotional distance. The food, the alcohol, the dead-end relationships—I turned to all those things because I didn't value myself; I hurt a lot of people, but I especially hurt myself. It was shame that kept me disconnected all that time—from myself and from God.

One of the many special problems of sexual abuse, perhaps the most destructive, is that the victim assumes the shame for what was done and then colludes with the abuser by covering it up. In the cruel twists and turns of that process, deep damage is done to the spirit. The extent of the damage plays a major role in how long it takes people to recover from it, why so many people never do recover from it, and why those who struggle to heal go through so many setbacks. I can only say that if sexual abuse has been your experience, the child in you who yearns to be reconnected will not relent until you heed its voice. When you do, you will experience the first of many floods of relief, rushes of joy, and stretches of serenity that reconnection will bring. Your innocence restored, you will become God's kid again.

Special Problems of Sexual Abuse

The Charm Factor

As my knowledge about sexual abuse grew and my healing began to make a significant difference in the way I looked, thought, and acted, I kept thinking more and more about my mother. I'd noticed there were certain patterns that could be observed in people who have been sexually abused. Years later, as I gave examples of these patterns at staff meetings, I realized the person I was describing was my mother. There were a lot of things about her I had never understood. One was a love–hate relationship she had with men. I started putting some things together in my mind. Then a light went on in my head. She had been abused by my grandfather, too.

I decided I had to ask my mother directly about what I suspected. When I did, she at once began to cry uncontrollably. She continued to cry and I continued to comfort her, but she could not talk about the incest. Days later she came to see me in a very emotional state and started to verbalize what had happened. The story poured out of her: Her mother had gone to the hospital to have her youngest brother, Eddie. While my grandmother was in the hospital, my grandfather had committed incest with my mother. Ever since, my mother had carried animosity for Eddie, because she associated the incest with his birth. Her treatment of Eddie had always caused me a lot of anguish. I loved my youngest uncle and thought he was a wonderful guy. When I was growing up, I even used to carry his picture around and sometimes told people he was my boyfriend. I could never square my perception of him with my mother's some-

103

times downright hatred. Now that Mom confronted her feelings, she decided to make amends with Eddie. When they came together and she explained what had happened to her, he understood her venomous anger that had been directed at him rather than at their charming and wonderful father. Although Eddie was shocked and sad, because he loved Poppa, he believed her.

Because of my own experience and that of countless others, I have become convinced that secrets are what make people sick, and burying them also keeps them stuck in their sickness. When writing my first book, *It's Not What You're Eating, It's What's Eating You,* I debated for a long time how much I should disclose about my personal life. On the one hand, being completely forthcoming and honest had been my direction from the beginning, and it had succeeded in helping people in ways I had never imagined. On the other hand, I worried about the effects on my family. I gave a copy of the manuscript to my uncle Eddie and asked him for his opinion. He laughed his big barrel laugh and said, "What's your mother going to say about this?" I guess he wasn't going to let me off the hook.

In the end, I decided to tell my story of incest because time and again I had seen how disclosure of an abuse, especially a long-held secret, has a great healing effect upon anyone who shares the experience. Some may respond with disgust or denial, but others may burst into tears of empathy and love. After a long debate with myself, I decided to disclose my secret.

After the book was published, two cousins contacted me and said they had also been sexually abused by my grandfather. They said because of the book they were finally convinced they aren't bad, that what happened to them was incest, and that they could begin to cope with the damage done to their sense of self. They are both on the mend. Another of my cousins complained about me, "How could Janet talk about the family like this?" I told my mother, "She can only say that because it didn't happen to her. If it happens to you, then you have a totally different perception."

My cousins' disclosures affected me in a weird way. I had always thought I was the only one, but it was apparent that my grandfather just went after all the young girls, that he felt he had a license to do whatever he wished, and with so many female grandchildren, he had himself a field day. "It wasn't him, it was the drink," was the attitude of the women in my family, passed from generation to generation. By blaming the abuse on the drink, we could lessen the discomfort of dealing with the wrong things my grandfather did and focus on the part of him that was charming and wonderful.

One day I was attending a workshop on the characteristics of the sex offender, and I heard a description of how perpetrators groom their victims. Suddenly I felt an incredible surge of anger. How dare he! I wanted to shout. The abuse was *not* just something that happened because of drink or a sudden urge.

Most people have a perception of sex offenders as the lurking stranger, someone seedy looking and evil. However, they are more likely to be charming and well loved. They consciously groom not only their victims, but everyone in their world into thinking they're wonderful, so they can get away with the abuse. It's the nature of human beings to overdevelop strengths in order to camouflage weaknesses. Just as victims overcompensate for their shame by their constant doing and people pleasing, perpetrators work very hard cultivating their image as a wonderful person. They win people over to assure their credibility if the abuse is ever detected.

Because everybody loves the perpetrator, the victim has a difficult time. Perception is fractured: How could someone so lovable do this to me? To this day, there are times when I am in conflict with myself over the two sides of my grandfather—the awful side and the wonderful side. I am inclined to believe that this is a common conflict, and I am learning to accept it as something that may never be resolved.

The more survivors of sexual abuse who tell me their stories, the more I hear about the perpetrator as a wonderful person who nobody can believe would do such a terrible thing. One woman I know well had given up ever being believed and, in fact, had learned to tolerate not being believed by just about everybody in her family and circle of friends. Years before I met her, she had discovered her husband sexually abused her daughter, an only child. The couple divorced because of it, even though she loved her husband very much. He was able to deny any wrongdoing very successfully.

When the word got out, not only did the husband's family defend him, so did the wife's family and all their mutual friends. He even convinced the court officer supervising his visitations that he was actually a great guy. As a result of her former husband's ability to charm, the woman lost the affection of friends, in-laws, and her own family and was blamed for doing a terrible thing to the man and to her daughter. She was completely isolated from the full and exciting life she once had.

Through all this severing of ties, the woman and her daughter remained close, but for years they never mentioned the father by name. They could have long reminiscences about an experience the three of them shared, but it was as if he had not been a part of it. The situation might have remained static indefinitely, except for the fact that the compulsion to sexually abuse was left untreated. The father, who had remarried, committed incest with his new daughter and, once again, was turned in. This time, unable to keep his image of "the wonderful guy" intact, he killed himself.

After he died, a healing process began to take place between the mother and the daughter. Not only could they grieve for him, they could talk about how he *was* a wonderful person and they could laugh, cry, and utter his name.

The dilemma of the charm factor is the ambiguity it creates in the victim. We start to reflect and think we were somehow responsible. We need very much to understand that we were not in any way responsible for any of the abuse. I know I found it most helpful to acknowledge how I was set up by my grandfather, how his abuse of me was a premeditated act, how I was manipulated by him to keep silent, and how calculated and unfair the relationship was! It didn't matter whether I talked or didn't talk about what he did. Whereas I was a confused child, he was an adult who knew exactly what he was doing. He worked around the clock at his only real job, being a wonderful fellow, who I am sure would have denied most convincingly anything I had tried to say. When I understood that, forgiving myself flowed right out.

(You may feel at this point that forgiveness is very far away. Maybe you have picked up this book because you're searching for something that will make you feel better about yourself. Maybe whatever previously worked for you to numb the pain of disconnection no longer works and in desperation you are turning to this or that remedy. Or you may be using something that still works and numbs the pain. The only trouble is, it is also numbing your spirit; it is numbing who you are. Whatever your need, if you have a desire to experience life deeper than you are, keep reading.)

As long as I kept my feelings of shame a secret, I was too numb to feel much of anything. Keeping the lid on my secret didn't allow me to experience sex, love, or intimacy with anyone. How could I? I was this terrible person who had no value. The only intensity I was able to experience was with the assistance of a distorter—food, alcohol, a good deed, an accomplishment—something outside of myself. The worst of it was that meaningful connection with others was impossible. I was disconnected from the greater part of myself, and I needed to bond myself together before I could bond with others.

If you truly want that reconnecting to happen, it will. That bonding is the wine of life. It's what makes the whole world exciting. It's the promise, the hope. Take the action and you will get there.

Sexually Abused Men

I have come to believe that as shameful as sexual abuse is for women, it's worse for men because it can shatter their sexual identity. Women don't feel "less than a woman" because of the abuse, but abused men have to cope with feeling "less than a man," as the following case history describes.

Two brothers, four years apart, were sexually abused for a five-year period during their late childhood and early adolescence by an older stepbrother. At the time, neither brother knew about the other's abuse. As adults, the younger brother became homophobic, and the other worried that he might be gay because he had sometimes experienced orgasms with his stepbrother.

The younger brother came into treatment first, but then the older brother followed after attending a very intense and healing family session. Although their defenses were powerful, eventually both were able to separate their sexual identity from the abuse. The younger brother has ceased being homophobic. He had never felt comfortable with these negative emotions he had had for gay people. Once he discovered the real source of his feeling, he was able to defuse his hatred. I often wonder how much homophobia has its roots in deeply repressed memories of sexual abuse.

The older brother had a more difficult recovery. Not until late in treatment was he able to deal with the pleasure aspect, which was what was bothering him the most. Fear about sexual identity is so threatening in sexually abused boys that the trauma is repressed even more deeply if there was pleasure involved. Any time we associate a negative action with pleasure we become confused in our brain, our body, our whole being.

Being Believed

I will never forget the period of obsession I went through after disclosing my long-kept secret. I wanted to talk about it to everybody. I had hidden it for years, and in a short time I was talking about it on national TV! I had the good fortune of being supported by a lot of people who did believe me, including close family members, and so many people were hungry for what I had to say because it shed light on their own history with this most sensitive of issues. I am constantly gratified by the feedback I receive that my disclosure has helped people and that hearing, not about the abuse but about what I did as a result of the abuse, has resonated in them and they no longer feel so alone. I know that all the courage I needed to tell my secret was worth it when someone tells me that I gave them the hope they desperately needed. Disclosure of the secret was twice blessed, for it also brought up my mother's secret to her great relief and our own mutual benefit. Now we can be real around each other.

However, not everyone is so fortunate; many people uncover their secret and are not believed. I heard of a psychotherapist whose response to a patient's disclosure had been, "Are you sure you didn't just dream it?" Some people react with a lot of denial and negative energy concerning sexual abuse. I remember one doctor exclaiming, "What's the big deal?"

Sometimes people are full of ambivalence and downright unwillingness to believe a secret they have discovered about themselves. I strongly recommend that until you have no further doubts about what happened that you contain the information to people who *do* have the ability to be supportive: a therapist, a member of the clergy, a sexual abuse center, or someone you sense is a caring individual who will understand and hear you out. Take a chance on someone you think might be a good person to talk to, and check out your feelings when you are in his or her presence. How does your body feel? Is the person giving you anything back that feels warm, supportive, or caring?

We need to be careful about whom we talk to, to

make sure there's some kind of bonding. In the early stages of discovery, it is not a good idea to share your secret with family members who you fear will not believe you or persons who love the abuser and won't want to believe you. IT'S IMPORTANT TO REMEMBER THE GOAL IS NOT TO BE BELIEVED; IT IS TO DIFFUSE YOUR SECRET BY TALKING ABOUT IT TO THE RIGHT PEOPLE SO IT WON'T BLOCK YOUR ENERGY ANYMORE.

The same discretion holds true outside the family. Most people don't know how to respond to a disclosure of sexual abuse, and if they fail to respond to it because they don't know what to say, we might interpret their silence as a message that there is something wrong with us. We don't need any more of that!

The fear of not being believed can keep you holding on to a secret that has damaged your life. It is a very real fear. Anyone who feels it is not being paranoid, for until quite recently, revelations of childhood sexual abuse were rare to nonexistent; speaking out was an act of courage very few people were willing to take.

I am very glad the subject of childhood sexual abuse is now out in the open where society as a whole must come to grips with it. Nevertheless, we need an overview of the recent past to understand just how profound a change has taken place, and why the new era of disclosure is so challenging and fraught with difficulty.

The Freudian Century

Early in the 1890s, Sigmund Freud treated eighteen patients, two-thirds of them women, for what was then called hysteria. Most of the patients were referrals by colleagues who diagnosed them as "untreatable liars." Freud soon became intrigued by the similarities among this random group. One similarity was how they experienced puberty: "A shrinking from sexuality, which normally plays some part at puberty, is raised to a high pitch and is permanently retained." In adulthood, the patients remained in that state of discomfort, "psychically inadequate to meet the demands of sexuality."

Another similarity was the presence of childhood sexual experiences, revealed to him with a great amount of resistance and anguish. Examining a patient's sexual life in puritanical nineteenth-century Austria was not regarded as reputable, but Freud took the risk. As a consequence, his practice suffered.

In his continued examination of the eighteen hysterics, Freud was struck by the power of their resistance to the memory of their traumas: "One gets the impression of a demon striving not to come to the light of day, because he knows that will be his end." By persistent dissolving of their resistance, eventually all eighteen patients told him the same story: of being sexually abused as a child, usually by a family member.

The stories were always told in the same heartwrenching manner, displaying the same disbelief and reluctance to reveal the vivid recollections that were flooding the patients' minds. Freud took note of the uniformity of detail in each revelation and the way

112

the patients minimized the most horrific events. He eloquently describes their anguish:

> Doubts about the genuineness of the infantile sexual scenes . . . and behavior of patients while they are reproducing these infantile experiences is . . . incompatible with assumption that the scenes are anything else than a reality which is being felt with distress and reproduced with great reluctance. Before they came for analysis the patients knew nothing about the scenes. They are indignant as a rule if we warn them that such scenes are going to emerge. Only the strongest compulsion of the treatment can induce them to embark on a reproduction. They suffer the most violent sensations, of which they are ashamed and try to conceal. [Even afterward] they still attempt to withhold belief, and emphasize they have no feeling of remembering the scenes. Why should patients assure me so emphatically of their unbelief, if what they want to discredit is something which . . . they themselves have invented?

Nevertheless, Freud did discredit his eighteen patients two years after presenting "The Etiology of Hysteria," or, as it is better known, "The Theory of Seduction," in which the above quotation appeared. In 1896, he presented his new theory before the Society of Psychiatry and Neurology in Vienna. Freud's "momentous discovery" of the childhood origins of hysteria was met with thunderous silence by his peers, followed by a period of total pariahhood. Freud had broken a code, the prevailing belief among the upper classes that incest was present only in the lower classes and had been bred out of "polite" society. Not one of his colleagues came forward to defend him.

Freud's retraction two years later was "The Theory of Infant Sexuality," a foundation of his life's work. He revised his previous theory of infantile seduction; it was now *a wish* to be seduced by the parent, not an actual seduction. On the rare occasions when he referred to his original theory, he called it his "far-reaching blunder." As for the eighteen patients, they returned to the category of "untreatable liar."

Imagine how many people in the past hundred years have been diagnosed as hysteric or otherwise but have actually been keeping the secret of abuse and searching for someone to believe them! It's too depressing to think about for long. However, I do want to focus on the continued influence of Freud on people in the mental health profession who are reluctant even today to believe what their patients tell them about sexual abuse. There are still professionals out there today who doubt the reality of their patients' stories of abuse and try to convince them that these awful things they suddenly remember or dream about—no matter how hurtful and degrading—are actually a wishful fantasy. I can't describe how much harm this can cause in doubtful, shame-based people searching for the truth about themselves.

Another difficulty in being believed has to do with the delay factor. In one poll taken after the Clarence Thomas hearings, 75 percent of those responding did not believe Anita Hill's allegations about Thomas's sexual harassment. The main reason they gave for not believing her was the delay factor: "If it happened, why did she wait so long before she said anything?"

According to that logic, an undiscovered secret loses credibility as time goes by. However, the impact that secret has on the person who represses it is never diminished. In fact, the longer the secret remains buried, the deeper the scars run. Defensive emotional barriers may protect us from painful memories, but they also disconnect us from our spirit. Healing can only happen when the layers of defense have been scraped away, the secret exposed, and its energy defused. How long that process takes has nothing to do with whether an act of abuse happened or not. To the contrary, the extent of the delay often has to do with the extent of the damage you have undergone and how much of your core being is shame.

Sexual Abuse in Families: A Moral Epidemic

Health care professionals have found that a high percentage of sexual abusers have themselves been sexually abused. It would seem that the act of having been violated is twisted in the victim's mind into the right to violate others. Once a sexual boundary has been crossed, it's as if the Golden Rule had been perverted into "Do unto others as you have been done unto." Within sexually dysfunctional families, there is a strong belief, on the part of the abused and abuser, that there is *nothing wrong* with repeating the abuse on another, less powerful family member. The victims' concept of right and wrong becomes clouded, leaving a murky area where they are also free to abuse a weaker family member and, like the offender, do so without empathy for their victims.

In some families there seems to be a tradition of sexual abuse as a secret privilege bestowed upon certain family members. That was true of my grandfather, who seemed to believe it was his prerogative to abuse the young female family members and never gave evidence of feeling any guilt or shame. One successful woman in her mid-thirties, a lawyer and the youngest of eight, confronted her father, the head of a prominent Chicago law firm, and told him that two of her brothers had sexually abused her when she was little. He waved his hand and replied, "Oh, well, boys will be boys."

The Assault of Knowledge: Abuse Without Touching

Many go through treatment having trouble defining themselves as survivors of sexual abuse because what happened to them involved no actual touching, but rather a lot of premature exposure to adult sexuality. The "let it all hang out" era of the sixties and early seventies gave rise to a time of free love and overt sexuality. Many people, now in their twenties and early thirties, report that their parents' nudity or openness about their sexuality troubled them. What should have remained a mystery to be discovered and enjoyed at a future time was too overwhelming and confusing for young minds. As a result, many children carried this uncomfortableness with sex into adulthood.

One woman in her mid-twenties recalls her early childhood as an exciting time when both parents worked at home and shared communal responsibility for a nursery school in the neighborhood. There the parents took very seriously their task of creating an environment that was free of the gender roles that could twist the developing mind of a child. Nevertheless, her parents' free-spirited ideas about nudity, particularly the father's exhibitionism, were disturbing to her little-girl mind. A sexual boundary had been crossed, and the impact on the child was the same as for one who had been molested—disconnection. Trying to make distinctions in how that disconnection happens is like calling an assault by a frying pan "frying pan abuse." Focusing on what happened rather than how you protected yourself in reaction to it only delays the discovery process. Don't let yourself get stalled there for too long.

Let Your Body Decide

Rather than search for a therapist to believe in your story, search for a therapist who believes in *you*, and conduct your search with a lot of careful consideration.

To take the mystery out of your search, pay attention to your body in the presence of a therapist at an initial visit. If your posture is closed; your legs and arms crossed; you are leaning back and have trouble making eye contact; or you feel ashamed, insecure, or "less than," find someone else to help you. You're not looking for a therapist who will impress you or make you feel uneasy. You are looking for someone you can feel safe around, and your body is excellent at communicating your instinctual response to people.

If the therapist seems nice enough but you do not feel you are getting something back, not necessarily in words but a feeling of support and positive energy, keep looking. If the therapist is full of enthusiasm and good words but you are not convinced it's for real, or if after a few visits you find your therapist is slow on the uptake and still not picking up the basic facts of your situation, keep looking for the good energy you need.

People who have been sexually abused have a special need for therapists who trust their instincts and intuition, take risks, and are actively involved in the process of recovery. Worst for us is the no-response approach (or, as I heard it recently described, to roars of laughter by a group of professionals, "the therapist as cadaver"). *We* have had enough problems with silence in our lives! *We* need responsive treatment: reality oriented and nurturing, but tenacious and insistent, by therapists who know about being stuck, value our lives even when we don't, and urge us to take action to solve our immediate problems while we probe into the past.

Avoid a therapist who in any way expresses doubt in your experience. There are those who would still cling to the Freudian view that people in polite society just don't do that sort of thing to children. Recently I heard some therapists at a conference discuss how sexual abuse was the "in thing" right now. "I don't know whether to believe my patients or wonder whether they've just picked up on the fad," said one.

Such a therapist might sit there and smile reassuringly and never give you a verbal clue, but your body will give you clues aplenty to let you know whether you are in the presence of someone who will believe in you, support you, and help you get into long-term recovery. If your body responds by relaxing its tension, if you find yourself leaning forward, gesticulating a lot, laughing a lot, talking a lot, and especially if you find tears come from out of nowhere and it feels good to shed them, grab that therapist. You may have found someone who, with the passage of time, you may learn to deeply trust. With the right therapist, you can work through anything. I have met many of these tough-but-tender nurturers over the years. Many of them are survivors of sexual abuse themselves, which they often say allows them to intuit a secret long before a patient is ready to grapple with it.

To me, seeking professional help for childhood sexual abuse is as necessary as seeking professional help for a major bodily injury. Survivors have undergone spiritual trauma, a shattering of their core identity and the loss of 60 percent of themselves. That's major!

In the absence of a therapist, do justice to yourself and join a support group. Start talking about it and look for good energy. There are also a growing number of twelve-step groups for incest survivors that are highly individualistic in their approach to recovery. Avoid groups where a great deal of the focus is on graphic details of the abuse or where anger and hatred predominate, particularly a hatred of men as a gender. Look for a group that is gentle as well as angry, and loving as well as accepting, one that focuses on recovery today rather than the horrors of the past.

Breaking the Last Taboo

When I wrote about my grandfather's incest in my first book, *It's Not What You're Eating, It's What's Eating You,* the taboo of disclosing the fact that you had been sexually abused was still very much in place. That was only five years ago. Today, the subject of incest has come out of the closet and is headline news. What a difference five years have made and who would have known how healing the new openness could be. It is amazing to me how healing the simple telling of the truth is among people who hold secrets. It's as if the hidden part of us wants so desperately to get reconnected that it will jump out at the first opportunity to be recognized. I have lost count of the number of people who have come into treatment after seeing the movie *Prince of Tides* with its graphic and disturbing flashback of a repressed memory of a violent rape.

I for one am very glad that the double taboo—an offense committed in secret and covered up by the victim—has at last been broken. Victims who keep silent should realize that perpetrators see that silence as vindication, allowing them to continue deceiving themselves that the victims "asked for it." The more people who refuse to be part of the coverup, the healthier we will become. Of course, no offender will thank us for our openness, and families in denial will fight back. Nevertheless, it has been my experience over and over that disclosure helps other survivors. Speaking the words out loud goes a long way to defuse the power of a long-held secret. The more people who come forward, the less filled with shame, fear, and isolation the rest of us will feel. Those still in denial will begin to realize they have been mistaken about what they had told themselves was unthinkable. Unfortunately, sexual abuse is thinkable, and it is commonplace.

This rapid change in perception has already changed the legal statutes regarding childhood sexual abuse in twenty-one states as of this writing, and bills have been introduced in the state legislatures of many others. Because of the delay factor, statutes of limitations in sex abuse cases have been extended, allowing victims to prosecute after memories resurface.

Every week there is a new story about sexual abuse among religious orders. Often, when such cases go to court, other victims come forward. The sexual harassment of women in the military is also being officially recognized, and women across the country ran for public office in the 1992 elections as a result of getting angry at the way Anita Hill was treated at her all-male Senate inquiry. Nearly every week there is a television news special or drama about this subject that has everyone so angry, fearful, and confused. Although a backlash has already set in, I think it's safe to say that nothing lasts forever, not even the well-kept, toxic secret of sexual abuse.

ACTIVITIES
Days 19-31

Day 19: Blow Up a Self-Poster

Find a photograph of yourself as a child that you like. Maybe you are all dressed up in your holiday clothes, surrounded by loved ones at a table, full of anticipation by a gift-laden Christmas tree, or about to blow out birthday candles. In other words, choose a photograph where you are full of your spirit. If you can't find a photograph, look for a child in a magazine who looks as you might have at that age or with whose eager little face you identify.

Take the photograph to a photocopy store and get it enlarged to a 14×18-inch poster. Roll up this slightly fuzzy poster of your spirit, take it home, and hang it on a wall in your safe place. Entitle it "My 60 percent."

Day 20: Time Line

Take a large sheet of wrapping paper and spread it on the floor or a table. Draw a horizontal line across the middle of the paper. This line represents your life, beginning with your birth at the left-hand margin of the paper. On this line you will illustrate your life up to the present. Leave the last one-third of the paper blank to represent the future. Using sketches, meaningful symbols, words, or a combination thereof, document the five most important events in your life—the ones that shaped the direction it has taken, beginning with your birth. Move on to your adolescence and adult life. If you can't keep the significant events to five, illustrate more. This activity is meant to be ongoing.

When you are through with your time line for today, roll up the paper and tuck it away somewhere in your safe place. You may find yourself going back to this document as time goes by and your perspective keeps changing. You may not be ready to depict the most significant events of certain periods of your life, particularly the recent ones where the dust hasn't settled yet. As you go through the ninety days, you may want to fill in some of the gaps in your life line and add important events as you remember them.

For today, select a particular event from the time line and write about it in your journal as if you were writing the story for someone who is unfamiliar with your background and culture. Describe this significant time in your life with as much sensory detail as you can, and tell how it has affected you or continues to affect you today.

Day 21: Foot Talk

Walking barefoot was one of the ways you intensely experienced the world as a child, for the bottoms of the feet are highly sensitive. You may have a certain sensation that comes to mind as you think about yourself as a barefoot child—of walking through fine dirt, breaking up clods of dirt in a freshly plowed field, the joy of squishing your toes in mud, or of walking barefoot over freshly mown grass or in sand along the shore. Did the child in you love to jump barefoot from rock to rock crossing a stream? Or gingerly tiptoe over a gravel driveway? Or sink heel and toe into the softness of melting asphalt?

This may not be the season for walking barefoot, but if it is, take off your shoes and feel the earth beneath your feet at the next opportunity. In the meantime, write in your journal about your favorite barefoot experiences as a child.

Day 22: Breathwork

When people get stuck, they have a tendency to go into hollow breathing: They compress rather then expand. The way they breathe is the way they connect, and it really expresses how they respond to everything that is happening. You may be completely unaware of your breathing. If that is the case with you, in times of stress it is particularly necessary for you to tell yourself to breathe, because just when your mind and body need the energy the most, you may be holding your breath! That's like revving the engine with no gas in the tank.

The next time you feel stressed out, check your breathing. Begin breathing from the stomach and the chest, and you may find some instant relief after a dozen deep breaths or so.

Initially, deep breathing needs to be a conscious effort. After a while, you will be able to do it without thinking. Deep breathing is difficult for many people because of fear or enculturation. It means expanding their chest, which they may protectively contract because it has such strong sexual connections. Many women have trouble breathing from the chest because they think their breasts are too big or they are unhappy with the way they are shaped. Deep breathing also means extending the belly, which we are constantly told to "suck in" as if being judged in a perpetual bathing suit competition in a beauty contest.

To get in the habit of deep breathing, do this activity until it becomes something you do voluntarily and ritually without conscious thought:

Lie on your back on your bed and place one hand on your chest. Place the other hand on your stomach. Expand first your stomach and then your chest as you take a slow, deep inhalation. You will know if both belly and chest are expanding if your breathing elevates them. When you can't comfortably take in more air, blow it out of your mouth, making a sound by pursing your lips together. This way you will be able to hear if you are exhaling through your mouth. Between breaths, let go of all your muscles and rest.

By the twelfth belly breath, you may be feeling light-headed. Stop the conscious slowing of your breath and simply be aware of the way your belly and chest rise and fall. Be conscious of the bellows effect of your lungs, a marvelous engineering construction. Be conscious of your heart beating under your hand; be aware of its steady pace. Lie for a while, marveling at all your body parts at work so wonderfully, unseen under your skin. Then slowly come to your knees; rise carefully (your brain is unused to such a hit of oxygen!); and, after you have grounded yourself, give your arms, legs, head, shoulders, hips, torso—the works—a very excellent rock-and-roll shakeout.

This belly breathing exercise, which takes just a few minutes, is a very good thing, too, when you are stressed out and need a pick-me-up. If you do it in bed when you have trouble falling asleep, you probably won't get past a dozen breaths before you're off to dreamland. If you don't want to fall asleep because you are preparing yourself for some memory work, lie comfortably on the floor, not in bed.

Day 23: Breathwork—Blockage

Complete the exercise for Day Twenty-two, breathwork, and after having taken twelve deep breaths, continue to breathe deeply but let go of your conscious control. Turn your attention to your body. Listen to it. Often, memories of events are stored in energy centers and express themselves as a knot in the stomach, a pain in the back or neck, or a stiffness in the jaw. In your mind, take an inventory of your entire body and check for knots and clinches and other stress indicators. If you feel pain anywhere, ask your body what the trouble is.

Breathwork can result in quite profound emotional unfolding. As you relax your body and release energy that has been blocked by stress, repressed feelings and memories may come tumbling out. Acknowledge them for what they are but know that they will pass and that your body has been relieved of the task of concealing them.

DAYS 24-28

The following five activities are constructed to increase access to traumatic memories. If you feel these activities don't apply to you, you may instead do five days of journal writing. Set aside three minutes each day and write in your journal for that time, keeping your pen in constant motion on the paper for the entire three minutes. If you find nothing to write, write the words "Nothing comes to mind I don't know what the hell I'm doing this for, etc." until something does come to you. At the end of the three minutes, read what you have written out loud.

You can resume the activities at Day Twenty-nine.

Day 24: Body Image

The purpose of this activity is to discover where in your body you store your emotions. Turn the lights low and play some soothing music. Notice how you are feeling in your body right now.

Scan your body to discover where you store your emotions.

Imagine a situation where you felt emotion and then noticed where in your body you experienced that feeling.

Where in your body does your ANGER reside?

Where in your body does your LOVE reside?

Where in your body does your GUILT reside?

Where in your body does your SHAME reside?

Where in your body does your FEAR reside?

Where in your body does your MOTHER reside?

Where in your body does your FATHER reside?

Where in your body does your JOY reside?

What have you learned about your body and your emotions?

What are you willing to change to give your body a rest?

Shut out of your mind what *others* say or think about your body image and mold what *you* believe your image to be.

Begin to pay attention to your breathing, simply noticing how this happens for you. Don't try to change your breathing pattern, but rather trust that, after all these years, your breath knows how to breathe itself. Just breathe naturally and notice:

What parts of your body move when you breathe?

In what order are they moving?

Are you breathing through your mouth or through your nose?

Are you inhaling all the way, or is there some restriction that prevents you from taking a full inhale?

When you exhale, do you empty your lungs completely?

Follow your breath and use it as a means to getting to know the inner areas of your body. Try to sense how much of the surface of your body is present in your awareness. Scan your surface to discover which areas of your body's surface are clear and which are vague or missing entirely from your awareness.

At the close of this meditation, perform some light-hearted activity or engage in a pleasurable distraction.

Day 25: Restimulation of the Trauma— Let the Body Talk

The purpose of this activity is to bring up significant memories. It should be preceded by the deep breathing or the progressive relaxation exercises.

Often feelings are locked in your body and you need to look for little clues. Lying in a relaxed state, ask yourself if a part of your body could talk, what would it say? For example, "I am Mary's arm. I have to push people away because they are hurting me."

If the part of your body couldn't talk, but could only make a sound, what sound would it make? Add a movement to accompany the sound.

Now address the body part, first as if you were the age when the trauma occurred and again in the present moment. What does it say to you?

If memories come up, welcome them. They are clues and guides to your recovery from trauma.

Day 26: Accessing Traumatic Memories— Giving Permission

Sit, facing an empty chair, and talk to your memory of a possible traumatic event and give it permission to emerge and sit with you.

Allow the memory to come forth. If there are any sights, sounds, or smells, give them permission to come and sit in the empty chair. Give them a shape and color and talk to them.

If there are significant people who might be able to fill in distant, vague, or painful memories, invite them to sit in the chair and talk to you.

Remember this: Burying the trauma is harmful, for it will emerge in one form or another. Remembering will *not* be as painful as the actual trauma. Remembering and acknowledging is the key to *releasing* the pain.

Day 27: Accessing Traumatic Memories— The Memory Box

The following guided imagery might be helpful in getting in touch with traumatic memories. Close your eyes and relax.

Imagine you are in a safe place. You go through a doorway and enter a room where you become aware of a big box that contains memories that you have locked up for a long time. You are aware of the box's size, shape, color, and what it's made of. You know the box contains your painful memories, but you are not afraid. You know that it is safe to remember. You look around the room and find a key that will open the memory box.

You open the box and find a photo album containing pictures of the painful experiences you have had. You allow yourself to reexperience the pain. You breathe deeply and know that you are okay. There are several photos that are faded. These are distant memories, but you allow them to become clearer and clearer. Look at the pictures and don't be afraid.

Open your eyes and process your feelings in your journal.

At the close of this activity, find something light-hearted to do. I recommend the simplest and most readily available distraction: Turn on a radio or TV until you find some music. Sing to it or, better yet, dance to it. This may seem like a corny thing to do after such serious business, but it's important to realize you can't take yourself out on an emotional limb and then just leave yourself there. You need to program in some balance, which is what a light-hearted closure to any memory access work will provide.

Day 28: What Was Missing?—A Guided Imagery

This activity is designed to help you focus on your nonsexual needs as a way of enhancing your sexual relationships. Dim the lights and play some soft music. Begin by doing some deep breathing. Then recall any sexual experience you have had that you consider typical. Remember where you were. What did the place look like? What were the sounds? What were the colors? What were the smells? What were you feeling? Notice how your body is reacting. Let your body, your spirit, your soul, your heart, be aware of the effects of the sexual experience. Now give yourself permission to remember what was missing.

What were you feeling? What were your needs? How did the experience affect you then? How does it affect you today? What were your fears?

Process these feelings in your journal.

Day 29: Restoring the Divinity of the Body

Survivors of sexual abuse have difficulty with sexual pleasure because long ago the sanctity of that experience was betrayed. Since then, their perception of pleasure has been twisted: They fear too much pleasure; they don't believe they deserve it; they don't think they can contain the pleasure; and they feel betrayed by their bodies.

The survivor of sexual abuse needs to make a gesture to turn that betrayal around. Our bodies did not betray us; *our bodies were betrayed*. Make up a regular cleansing ritual of your own choosing to wash yourself clean of all responsibility for that betrayal. As you let the water run over your skin and as you rub the skin with soap, tell yourself what you are doing: that you are cleansing your body of the betrayal and restoring your divinity.

Those who have not been sexually abused can also benefit from a ritual cleansing, for the divinity of our bodies is betrayed every day by advertisers who would demean us in order to get us to buy something to enhance our desirability. Because we are constantly bombarded with these negative messages, we need to do a regular ritual cleansing to acknowledge our real selves in all our real beauty, washed clean of the need to resemble a stereotype of someone else's choosing. I truly believe this type of betrayal is even more insidious than physical abuse in its ability to undermine our self-love and self-esteem, because we fail to see the extent of the damage it does.

Day 30: Ocean Meditation

If you live by the ocean, know that standing on the shoreline and looking out has a way of evoking repressed memories. I'm not sure why this is, but the pull of the waves and their breaking on the shore may have something to do with it.

If you cannot get to the coastline, it is possible to stand by the ocean in your mind and imagine the waves are very high and crashing all around you. Look to the horizon. As you continue to gaze far away, the waves start to calm down until they are just ripples that gently splash upon the sand. As the water calms, you are able to see into its depths and explore its hidden mystery; you can feel its quieting underwater peace. Sometimes the surface of the water becomes disturbed and choppy again, but in time the waves become ripples and roll away. Beneath the surface, the ocean remains peaceful and calm and full of hidden beauty. Feel safe and know that it's safe to feel.

Day 31: Meeting a New-Found Friend

This is a guided imagery to the discovery of hidden secrets and to the reconnection with your spirit. Because it is long, you might get someone to read it to you, or you can read it into a tape recorder and play it back. Allow yourself plenty of time. Play some soft and relaxing music, dim the lights, and prepare yourself for the journey by doing some deep breathing.

We will be going on a journey to a place that you've needed to go to for a long time. It's important that you feel relaxed and safe right now and that you allow yourself the permission and the freedom to experience all that is about to happen.

Pay attention to your breathing and begin to slow it down. Allow your body to become comfortable and relaxed. Tell yourself that you are in a safe place and are protected by all that is good, all that is peace, and all that is love. Know that you are a person seeking to improve the quality of your life and your relationships with the world.

Imagine that you are breathing in light and energy. As you breathe out, breathe out all of your anxiety and fear. Let them be exhaled. As you breathe in, allow the light and the energy to fill those spaces left behind. Allow the light and the energy to travel around your body, calming those parts that need to be calm. Fill yourself with light, power, love, and peace. You feel wise.

As you continue to slow your breathing down, you feel your body become lighter and lighter as if you could almost float. Continue to breathe in light and safety and breathe out tension. Imagine your body floating up. Your body begins to leave the room, and it floats up into the air as you continue to breathe in the light and energy, the safety, and the peace.

You feel your body floating up into the clouds. Now your body is floating up into the stars and now through the stars—higher, higher. Allow yourself to experience the freedom of your body floating. As you continue to float, know that we are going to go on a journey together. Allow yourself the permission to experience all that is about to happen. Know that you are protected.

Begin to feel your body float downward, back through the stars, now through the clouds and through the air, and finally, slowly, softly, you reach the ground. You feel the ground beneath your body, against your skin. You feel the clothes against your skin. You feel the air against your skin. The sounds in the background and the smells, and the energy—experience all that is around you right now and know that you are in a very special place where you need to be.

Now, in your mind, begin to sit up. Look around and see what is there. Stand up and feel the ground beneath your feet as you begin to move.

Feel the safety, the peace, and the serenity of being loved in this special place that you have allowed yourself to go to. As you walk along, you see the opening of a cave up ahead. As you walk closer to the cave, you decide to go inside. You are at the opening of the cave. You walk through and feel the change in temperature and the texture of the air, and you feel the walls of the cave with your hands.

It becomes dark and cold, and the sounds and smells are different. You may feel some fear and anxiety. Breathe out those feelings and breathe in the power of the energy and the light to replace them. Know you are safe and protected.

Now begin to walk into the cave deeper and deeper, safe in the knowledge that you are here because you need to be. As you move along the cave, you see something at the back of the cave and you're not sure what it is. As you move closer, it appears to be a person. As you continue to move closer, you see that figure is a child, rolled up in a ball, frightened and alone, angry, afraid, and tired. You move closer and see the child's clothes are torn; the child's skin is dirty. The child slowly turns its head and looks at you, and your eyes connect. The child begins to speak to you with its eyes, and you listen with your heart. Hear what the child is saying. As you move closer, look into the child's eyes and know that the child is you.

The child begins to speak to you. Listen to what the child is saying. Know that this little kid has been here a long time, waiting alone, frightened, angry, and sad.

You slowly reach out for the child's hand and the child is afraid. Then the child reaches its hand out toward you, and you feel that hand slowly slip into yours. As you gently pull the child toward you, it stands. You pick the child up and hold it in your arms. The child responds, and its body relaxes. Feel the body of the child against yours. Experience the excitement of the reunion and the joy of the safety and relief the child now feels. The child slowly turns its face toward yours and looks into your eyes. The child asks, "Why are you here?" Listen to the answers in your heart. The child now asks you another question, "Where have you been? Why did you leave me here all alone?" Allow yourself to experience all that you are feeling now as the child looks into your eyes.

You see the light at the opening of the cave, and you feel its invitation. You feel the child's happiness and excitement as you move closer and closer to the opening of the cave. Now that you've made your decision to leave, you begin to move more quickly toward the opening. You now begin to run and feel that child cling tighter to your body. You are there for the child, and the child knows it. As you run toward the opening of the cave, you feel a fresh wind blowing through your hair, against your skin. You feel the ground beneath your feet. You feel the light at the end of the cave as you see the opening of the cave become bigger and bigger. Now you are in the opening of the cave, and you stop and look around and the child looks around with you. As you look at the child's face, you see a smile and a sparkle in its eyes. You see happiness, joy, and freedom in the child's face.

You set the child down, and it begins to walk toward the sunlight where there is a beautiful meadow green with hay. The child invites you to come, too. The child tells you it has a gift for you and wants to whisper what it is in your ear. You bend down. The child whispers to you that it is giving you your spirit. Then it runs away from you and wants to play. You feel such joy in your heart to be given such an unexpected gift. You and the child laugh and roll in the meadow. You run and jump and play. You feel the freedom from all the shame and anger that has bound you.

As you play, you look around and the child is gone. At first you may feel afraid or sad, but then you realize the child is not gone. The child is in you, where it has always been. You feel the peace in the knowledge of that. As long as you allow yourself the permission to be that child, to experience that child, you can be in this place any time you want to.

As you walk along, enjoy the happiness and connection with your newfound friend, your spirit!

IV

Forgiving Yourself

Like everything else about recovery, forgiveness is a process. It doesn't suddenly happen that one day you are able to forgive, but gradually the burden becomes lighter until one day you realize you are no longer connected to the one who abused you, for forgiveness breaks that connection. If you don't forgive, you remain connected to the abuse. Forgive and you are reconnected with your spirit. That choice is a great motivator.

The reason why this chapter is called "Forgiving Yourself" is to alleviate any doubt that forgiving an offender is required in the process. Forgiving ourselves is the focus, because, as food addicts, we took our rage and loathing and transferred those bad feelings from the abuse to our bodies. The process of forgiveness can be broken down into three steps. First, you face it, acknowledging the secret and the feelings surrounding it. Second, you trace it, acknowledging the profound impact it has had on your life and your capacity to experience joy. Third, you erase it, a process that takes away the negative energy surrounding the secret.

Face It

The first time I really owned up to my grandfather's abuse was in the treatment center group discussing secrets. Because of my ability to dissociate, I had never truly understood what had happened to me. I kept the feelings around the abuse from emerging so I could cope. In the group, however, when I had to read aloud someone else's secret (which also happened to be about abuse), the feelings really started coming up. My whole body trembled, and my palms were wet. You will know you are truly facing something when you experience the unexpressed feelings your body has been storing all these years. It is a decision your body, not your mind, makes when the time comes.

At the conclusion of this chapter are exercises for facing a secret. The difficulty lies not in what actually happened, but in acknowledging all the time and energy that went into hiding it. This acknowledgment involves much more than people without secrets can ever comprehend. "Snap out of it," they say, but when your life once depended on *not* facing a fact, it is very difficult to make an abrupt turnaround and change ingrained patterns of behavior. Such an act requires an enormous amount of courage and a small amount of faith. It can only happen in a safe and structured setting, when a person is far enough along in recovery to meet the issues with self-love and self-trust.

Trace It

A patient of mine had a recurring dream of trying to move forward while being held back by an unknown force. In her dream she was trying to move along a sidewalk but couldn't get anywhere. In desperation, she grabbed at the cracks in the pavement and tried to pull herself ahead with all her might, but her body was a dead weight. Through therapy she realized these recurring dreams represented her resistance to trace her abuse; she was holding herself back in her recovery.

Then one night she had a breakthrough dream that she recorded in the notebook she left open by her bed. It was a most vivid dream, a variation on the recurring theme of not being able to move forward. This time she was back in her hometown (she could recognize local landmarks) and was trying to make her way to her childhood home, but she wasn't using the cracks in the sidewalk. In this dream she had to penetrate a bramble of knee-high weeds so tangled that she couldn't possibly make her way through them. No matter how hard she tried, she couldn't move. She even turned around and tried to push herself backward through them. She simply couldn't get through those tangled weeds. The feeling of being held back exhausted her and filled her with a familiar despair until a voice asked her, "Why do you have to go through them? Why can't you go over them?"

Tracing the abuse does not involve a reliving of

the incident; you don't have to dredge up the awful memories and suffer through them again. Tracing is not going *through*, but going *over* what happened, looking beyond the abuse itself to the impact it has had on your life.

For instance, until I talked about my secret, I had no understanding of the way I really felt about myself, especially concerning my repulsion and loathing at the idea of having sex.

In tracing the incest, I perceived myself in a new light as someone strong and trustworthy, a fighter who didn't understand that sex was not supposed to be a battle. I realized that my patterns of behavior with men were a direct result of the early sexual messages I received. My grandfather's abuse and my mother's warnings against men confused me. I developed my attitudes about sex and acted the way I did to protect myself. I always thought there was something wrong with me, but the tracing helped me very much in reframing my vision of myself.

After tracing the impact incest has had on my adult life, I am now able to understand why I married so many times. Each husband became someone to protect me, but I could never tell him what he was protecting me from because *I* was in the dark about what was really bothering me. Then, when the relationship became too difficult to sustain, I walked away. I am full of conflicting feelings to this day over how many times just a word from me might have made my marriages work, but I couldn't negotiate. I couldn't express myself or make myself understood. How could I when I didn't understand myself? I had been in a situation as a child where I could not possibly win except by keeping silent and stuffing down what I couldn't handle and, in the end, walking away. In moments of high stress, when a relationship hung in the balance, keeping silent and eventually walking away is exactly what I did as an adult.

Because it reveals so much powerful information about a life and its problems, the process of tracing takes place a little at a time. Effects of the abuse become evident as you are ready to handle the information. For instance, it took a while before I traced the effect of the incest on my body image and my attitude about sex. From the onset of my womanhood, I felt so tainted, and my sexuality was a source of so much discomfort and even outright terror. I always thought that I was dirty and spoiled, that something was wrong with me. It was many years before I experienced sex that was pure and fun and full of love, and it was only after I traced my incest and stopped blaming myself for what was a natural response to a horrible experience.

The difficult part of tracing is that it sheds light on a lifetime of choices. Tracing can cause distress as you begin to comprehend how powerful an effect this heretofore unseen force, your secret, has had on the way you reacted to events in your life and to the people with whom you chose to seek intimacy.

It often becomes clear that the significant people in your life were chosen not out of love, but as an unconscious link to past abuse. I was finally able to trace how every man I loved had been chosen not for the unique person he was, but out of my need for protection. Because I was not protected from my grandfather's abuse, seeking protection—not connection—was the major unconscious motivator in all my love choices.

It is hard for people to deal with the idea that the major decisions in their lives were made not in response to the adult's ability to negotiate in a way that serves the self, but out of a child's fear and doubt that still lingers. However, tracing is a necessary part of the process. It is part of freeing yourself from your past and allowing yourself to live in the present. Knowing the strong pull of your unconscious motivations will make you more responsible about future choices.

Understanding the Offender

Many people become so fused with the abuser that they have no idea who abusers are as individuals: what kind of personality traits they share with other offenders, what motivates them, or how they live with what they have done. In other words, most victims are ignorant about the victimizer, and in that ignorance they continue to feel culpable for the offense. Were they to know the truth about the offender, they could not possibly assume that responsibility.

The purpose of examining the offender's behavior is not to try to justify or explain, but to see the abuse from the offender's perception. Understanding the offender will hopefully result in the realization that he or she did whatever it took to shift responsibility for the abuse onto the victim. Offenders have to convince themselves that they're not to blame. Even convicted offenders who admit to the abuse often maintain their defense, "it's not my fault."

During the past few decades, incarcerated sex offenders have been studied by many disciplines. The following little-known facts are a compilation of the findings of the studies conducted by psychologists, sociologists, and criminologists on people who sexually abuse. They are presented to assist you in understanding the way offenders distort reality in order to live with their guilt. Through that understanding, I hope you can let go of a lot of negative emotions and get on with the process of forgiving yourself.

1. *Offenders sexualize power.* One of the most striking conclusions these studies draw is that lust and desire are not what motivate the abuser. It is power, what Henry Kissinger once called "the ultimate aphrodisiac." The abuser is in a power relationship and sexualizes that power.

2. *The offender is completely lacking in empathy for the victim and blames the victim for the abuse.* People who sexually abuse children have narcissistic cores. They don't really see other people for who they are, but rather how they can be used. Others are not individuals but extensions of themselves, especially a spouse or children. Offenders don't experience guilt because they really believe that the victim belongs to them, and they feel entitled to do what they do. If they are caught offending, they feel guilty about getting caught, not about what they did.

3. *If victims do not protest, offenders can continue to believe that what they are doing is not wrong.* In the secrecy surrounding an act of sexual abuse, offenders are able to distort reality and even convince themselves that the child likes the abuse or somehow encourages it. If a child reaches an age where he or she begins to resist, the offender will go to great lengths, using manipulation and threats, in order to prolong the cover-up. At this point, the offender will often move on to a younger victim.

4. *Seventy to seventy-five percent of sex offenders studied reported being sexually abused in their own childhood.* The vast majority of offenders have lived their entire lives with distorted perceptions of reality and twisted beliefs; they themselves were victims of abuse. They are also disconnected and live in discomfort and despair, having to vigilantly play roles—Mr. Nice Guy, Mrs. Wonderful, the One Who Can Do No Wrong. It is why offenders work so hard at convincing themselves as well as their victims that they are blameless.

Sex offenders live in denial year after year. Their denial is so strong they can be caught in the act of abuse and refuse to admit that anything bad is happening. Their ability to deny makes them dangerous. Denial is especially strong in abused people who become abusers of their own children. They minimize the most horrific stories of their own abuse as children and apply the same perception to the way they treat their own kids: "It's not that bad."

5. *The sex offender will continue the abuse until treated.* Just as the dispirited survivor of childhood abuse remains lost on a crooked path until treated, unable to change, so does the one who abuses. The survivor has the small comfort of being the innocent party. For the offender, there is no comfort to be had anywhere except in denial.

Women—The Hidden Offenders

In one study of one thousand incestuous fathers, of the 70 percent who reported being sexually abused as children, 44 percent said the source of the abuse was the mother. In another study conducted on one hundred adults who had been sexually abused by their mothers, not a single man and only 3 percent of the women told anyone about the abuse. Their shame was so great that they kept the secret for years, all the while living with murderous and suicidal thoughts. Eighty percent reported that the abuse was "the most hidden aspect" of their lives. One must wonder if the statistical rarity of female offenders has less to do with the infrequency of such abuse and more to do with how much abuse by women is denied and suppressed.

Erase It: Forgiving Yourself

For hundreds of years, the special problem of sexual abuse has been the secrecy; people simply denied its existence, and those who insisted on knowing and revealing the truth about themselves were diagnosed as "incurable liars" or worse. Finally, however, the last taboo has been broken. I am grateful that no one has to suffer the burden of sexual abuse in isolation anymore, for its prevalence on all levels of society can no longer be denied. Pandora's box has been opened and its contents revealed to the public consciousness, and now, instead of a few people struggling in isolation, *everyone* is struggling with the subject of what is abuse and what can be done to detect and prevent it.

As I wrote this chapter and absorbed the impact of the research, I kept thinking about how I had carried the burden of my secret alone for so many years, never hearing or reading anything that could help me deal with it. Now I see how my story becomes part of a larger picture of the great numbers of us who have struggled in the same silence. The more I look at it and trace the lines and features, that picture is a story about the resilience of the human spirit. How amazing we are to be able to live with such a burden! However much we may have undergone at the hand of fate or an individual, we can free ourselves at any time. We can forgive ourselves.

One of the hallmarks of treatment is that when the healing of childhood wounds begins, our patients' repressed memories of having wounded others, especially their own children, begin to surface. These memories surface with a flood of guilt and remorse. We have to actively provide the patients with a lot of balance so they don't confuse legitimate remorse with the shame they're trying to get rid of. We have to help them distinguish between self-imposed undeserved shame and appropriate guilt.

During treatment, many victims see for the first time all the abuse they have inflicted upon themselves. Often, abused people become addicts, doing considerable damage to their bodies, minds, and spirits. Because they are so filled with shame and self-loathing, they feel justified in turning their buried anger inward.

Forgive yourself for all the harm you have done to yourself; it is the first step in breaking the cycle of abuse.

Letting In, Letting Go

I could not let go of the past until I was able to stop trying to understand what had happened. I persisted in trying to make sense out of the senseless. I kept trying to figure out how my grandfather could love me and still do what he did or how I could have continued to love him even though he hurt me. However, there was no sense in trying to understand.

I was confused. I had been in that confusion for so long, ever since the nuns would tell us, "God is going to protect you. He sees everything." Well, then, I used to wonder, if God sees everything, how come he doesn't protect me? Don't I matter? Decades later I was still beating my head against this wall of futile thinking, always looking for a reason why.

Forgiveness means letting go of your need to understand. It is about the 60 percent that is your spirit, not the 30 percent that is your cognitive self. Forgiveness means expressing your anger at its deepest, where it is about hurt and loss, and then letting it go. Although the anger is justified, it is still negative energy stored for too long, and it must be diffused. As the months went by after I disclosed my incest, I continued to obsess on it, burning with long-held anger for the damage my grandfather had done. However, I reached a point where I felt as if my anger took too much energy. I felt as if it was burning *me*. I had to let go of those feelings for my physical health and peace of mind.

In the process, I discovered that letting go didn't mean giving up anything. It wasn't a loss, for when I finally let go, I let in my spirit, from which I had been disconnected so long, and it filled me with energy and joy. The effects of letting in this spirit of mine were profound. Before, I was connected to my grandfather through the abuse. I persisted in obsessing on it, trying to understand, and it had a lot of negative power in my life. After I let my spirit in, the old thoughts that ran in my mind, the old confusion, self-doubt, and self-anger, were lifted from me. I felt so much happier!

I now have the power that once went into repressing all my feelings about the abuse and my fear and shame. And believe me, that is a lot of power. I could do something else with all that energy—live. I could accept everything that had happened so far and move forward.

Failing to forgive yourself will keep you stuck in the past. There is a story in the Bible about Lot's wife. She and her husband were fleeing the wicked cities of Sodom and Gomorrah, and God had warned them to hurry away and not look back. However, Lot's wife kept looking back until finally she was turned into a pillar of salt.

Not letting go can turn people into pillars of salt, a monument to all the tears they have shed. Letting go of a toxic past is the best thing anyone can do for themselves, for with it goes the pain, the sense of frustration and hopelessness, and the blasts of negative energy fueled by hate.

I stopped looking back. After a certain point, I realized craning my neck in that direction didn't help much in moving me forward. However, I have seen people who have been stalled in the forgiveness process until it has drained their lives of all happiness and hope. The whole point of forgiveness is to change the focus of attention from the past to the present, where we can begin to change the patterns that have failed us for so long and start living in the only moment that counts—now.

Today I believe I'm a better person for all I've gone through. I am able to acknowledge that the incest played a part in making me who I am, that because of it I know something about human nature that other people don't know. This acknowledgment has helped me reignite the spark of divinity that the incest had all but extinguished.

Maybe if I had had one of those nice, normal lives some people are supposed to have, I wouldn't have done anything with my life, taken on challenges, or tried so hard to prove that I'm worthy. Maybe I would have had impatience rather than empathy and encouragement for people who are stuck. Maybe I wouldn't have the passion I have for life now.

When I think back on what happened to me in my youth (which I hardly ever do and have thought more about it while writing this book than I ever have), I can now tell myself with assurance that while I didn't want these things to happen, they did all the same, and what I do with my life now is what matters, not what happened to me long ago. There's so much to do!

ACTIVITIES
Days 32-37

Day 32: Seventy Times Seven—Forgiving Yourself

In the Bible we are instructed to forgive our enemies, not once but seventy times seven. There seems to be some kind of significance to this formula, for it also works in forgiving yourself. A legal pad has thirty-five lines, which makes it a perfect choice for this activity. Write a message of forgiveness, such as "I forgive myself," on each line of both sides of the paper. Do the same to six more sheets of legal paper. You may wish to forgive yourself for specific things on some of the seven sheets.

Keep these seven sheets of paper near your bed. Read them every night for seven nights before you go to sleep so you can internalize the message. You may not believe it at first, but something happens during this process of writing and then reading the same message seventy times that gets you to self-forgiveness. It won't happen right away, and if you find you aren't reading the pages every night or that you are skimming over them rather than really focusing on the message, you are still having trouble letting go. What is standing in your way is your nemesis, shame, which needs more eradicating. Continue with the activity knowing that the process will work if you truly want to be free.

Day 33: A Letter from the Abuser

Although this reads as a simple assignment, it may result in an onrush of deeply buried feelings. Know in your heart that doing the activity can have enormous self-healing value.

Think over the people who have hurt you in your life and select one. Write a letter to yourself from that person, apologizing for the abuse and making amends. Read the letter aloud and then destroy it. If you are at a computer, you can use the delete function—destroying the evidence without a trace. Or you may want to make a ritual of burning, which is a very old rite of spiritual cleansing, or you can simply shred the letter into tiny pieces and flush it down the toilet. You might find your own method of disposal of all these bad feelings and the powerful negative energy around them. Process your feelings in your journal. After the activity, do something enjoyable for a while that does not involve eating—go to a movie, watch some comedy on television, listen to music, read a history book, novel, or the biography of someone you admire.

Day 34: A Reply

Write a reply to the letter you wrote yesterday. Let your feelings for the abuser flow; feel safe and allow yourself to write whatever comes to your mind. Don't think about what you are writing, just write it. Try to get it all out. There should be several paragraphs that begin with "And another thing . . ." before you close. It is important to describe how the abuse made you feel in your body, how it disconnected you from your spirit, and how that has affected your life.

Read the letter out loud. Give yourself time to process, acknowledge, experience, and express any feeling that may come up.

The purpose of your reply is to diffuse bad feelings. Negative energy has been inside you all these years. Now it has finally been discharged through your fingertips, briefly traced on the paper, and then transformed into nothingness. Do you feel the release?

You can destroy the letter or keep it in your safe place where you can read it at a future time when you may find yourself feeling unentitled to your anger and sense of loss.

Day 35: Forgiving Yourself—The Deepest Secret

The following guided imagery should be preceded by deep breathing or the progressive relaxation exercise (see Day Six, page 46). Allow plenty of time. Lie comfortably and close your eyes.

Imagine you are playing a videotape of the movie of your life. It is a private screening. Beginning with your earliest years, scan the story of your life for the scenes in which you were abused by someone, fast forwarding with the remote control button from scene to scene up to the present. Pay attention to how you feel when you watch these scenes.

Now take a moment to rewind the videocassette to the beginning and give the movie of your life a second screening, this time focusing on the scenes where you harmed others. How does watching the scenes make you feel? Describe those feelings out loud.

When you have taken in all you can, stand up and give your body an overall shake. If you feel particularly low, put on some music and dance before going on to the next part of the activity.

Now write yourself a letter forgiving yourself for the people in your life you have harmed. Describe how you could make amends without their knowledge. What could you do right now to discharge the guilt you feel for the damage you've done? For example, you might do a good deed for someone in memory of a person you harmed or send a contribution to a worthy cause he or she espoused. Or you might send a loving letter or something needed to someone you harmed just out of the blue for no reason. The point is to make *private* amends—to yourself more than to the other person—so that you can dissolve those guilty feelings before they activate your shame.

In the days to come, pay attention to how you feel. If you do not feel immeasurably better about yourself, you may need to do this activity again.

Day 36: Forgiveness—A Guided Imagery

Prepare yourself for this guided imagery by deep breathing and lie comfortably on the floor with your eyes closed. Envision your abuser as a very young child. Remember what we know about abusers: that they were likely to have been abused as children, too. Speak to the disconnected spirit of that child, words that the child is yearning to hear but never did. Envision your abuser having the courage to forgive him- or herself for what he or she has done. Feel the healing effect that would have on the abuser and on you. Know you have been healed by it just by envisioning its possibility.

At the close of this activity, do something joyful that does not involve eating.

Day 37: Forgiveness Meditation

Read the following statements about forgiveness out loud. Then close your eyes and let your mind become still. Welcome the emergence of new perceptions. You may want to read this meditation nightly while you work on letting go or copy it in your journal. You may want to add some thoughts about what forgiveness means to you. Exactly what good things would come about if you let go?

- Forgiveness is not the denial of a wrongdoing. It frees ourselves, not the offender, from all responsibility for the abuse.
- Forgiveness means I give up the victim role in all its familiarity and occasional payoffs.
- Forgiveness means I give up the power to inflict guilt and to seek vengeance
- Forgiveness breaks the tie that binds me to the offender.
- Forgiveness brings the peace I have always been seeking.
- Forgiveness emancipates my spirit from my prison of shame.
- Forgiveness connects and bonds me to my spirit. I forgive to set that spirit free.
- I forgive.

V

Recovery

Life is a banquet and most people are starving.
—from *Auntie Mame,*
by Patrick Dennis

The 60 Percent

After I had gone through the process of forgiveness,
it took some time, but soon my core of shame was
gone and with it that overwhelming feeling of gloom
and doom about my body that had been with me ever
since I could remember. I began to feel lighter inside,
more buoyant, like a weight had been lifted from me.
Gradually I began to feel a new kind of energy—not
the desperate energy that drove me to do things to
hide my shame or the energy of rage that burned in
me after I disclosed my secret. This new energy was
a steady supply that surged through me efficiently
and purposefully to benefit myself as well as others,
and it felt good.

One day, two years after disclosing my secret, I

went to Seattle to lead a retreat. I can remember every detail of a certain moment of that trip: I had gone walking in the woods and found myself surrounded by a stand of majestic pine trees, their tips all pointing upward. As I craned my neck trying to figure out how tall they might be, I had a sense of my emerging spirit in the form of a deeply comforting knowledge that I was a good person. That knowledge grounded me like the trees rooted in the earth. I looked beyond the treetops to the sky, where there were slowly moving banks of the most beautiful pink-tinged clouds. My skin tingled, and I was flooded with a blend of delicious feelings. I didn't understand what was happening to me, but I felt it. There was the most wonderful smell of wood burning. I walked back to the campsite. Someone had built a fire and was roasting marshmallows. The fire crackled, and the birds sang the most beautiful song I'd ever heard. I felt so wonderfully alive, experiencing the world completely as I hadn't done in a long time.

The entire experience of that day in the woods is bathed in a halo of good feeling. It made me feel three-dimensional, aware how I was moving through time and space on this fascinating planet where one life will never be long enough to experience everything. I know that moment will always be with me, the shock of feeling reconnected to my spirit for the first time. Since that trip, there have been similar luminous moments and each one contained that spark of recognition, a kind of déjà vu that I believe comes from being reunited with that determined little dancing kid, God's kid, who was so insistently full of life and whose spirit fills me now.

I once watched the sun rise over Los Angeles and thought how the light from the streetlamps that stretched to the horizon were like the energy that once kept me going when I was in the dark about my secret. It was limited in how far it could illuminate, providing light but little warmth, and it cost a lot to keep the power going. However, the light from the rising sun was like being reconnected with my spirit: Little by little, it illuminates me, chasing away all shadows, and as it strengthens it warms and nurtures me, too, stimulating my growth. Before, nothing had seemed possible; now everything seems possible with this newfound energy.

During the early years of my recovery, my energy was astounding. I was like Arnold Schwarzenegger in my ability to take on anything that came my way. When I started college at the age of thirty-two, I was so heavy I had to sit on the floor because I couldn't fit into a desk, but my spirit urged me on, day after day, year after year. All through my early thirties, once the kids were in bed, I hit the books until midnight, slept six hours, then woke to work a part-time job before going to class.

I wasted no time on self-defeating behavior or doing for the wrong reasons. I knew exactly what I wanted to do with my life. All the past confusion about who I was and why I was here was gone. I knew my mission was to help people like myself get on and stay on the journey of recovery. For the first time, I knew who I really was.

Sometimes people approach early recovery thinking they have to start all over and create a new identity for themselves. That is not what happens at all. You don't have to create the Real You, for you already have been created. What you need to do is to evoke your spirit, which has spent many years in hiding, and call it by name. You need to define yourself not in terms of the world, but in terms of your newfound spirit and what that spirit values. Then, inevitable as the sunrise, in its own time and its own speed, it will come.

Recently a woman asked me to describe my spirit. I said at once, "Abundant, giving, caring." Afterward I thought about that word *abundant,* which came out of my mouth before I had time to consider my answer. I'd never used that word to describe myself, and yet it exactly defined my spirit. When a definition closely fits, it floods an internal emptiness. You may be in for a similar surprise when you try to define your spirit. I believe it is the only question we need to ask ourselves about who we really are. All the rest will follow, for your spirit is most eager for a chance at the wheel.

Do you know how I know my spirit is in the driver's seat? Lately I have noticed that when I travel, taxi drivers or hotel employees often ask me, "What are you so happy about?" Because I haven't said or done anything to evoke such a response, I know they are experiencing my spirit. The way I have defined that spirit has changed the way other people experience me. My spirit is just tickled pink to be in charge of my wonderful life.

Some people have so much spirit that they appear larger than life. How often have you heard someone talk about meeting a famous person and being surprised at how small he or she was? Take George Burns, for example, who is physically a very small man. He seems to occupy far more space than his physical presence because of his spirit. There is freedom and spontaneity in him; here is a man who loves his work and is willing just to be, and that makes him larger than life. He may be small in stature, but his spirit fills an entire room.

Conversely, when our spirit is repressed, we become smaller than life. People have a hard time getting a sense of who we are. We constrict. Many patients come into treatment holding back from the throat when they talk, as if they were trying to choke down their voice. They don't intend to let people experience their being; that would make them feel too vulnerable. Instead, they use whatever energy they have protecting and defending themselves.

When I was disconnected from my spirit, the only way I could find relief for my depression was through drinking. Alcohol used to be called spirits, and although it dulled the pain and probably saved my life by providing me with a false sense of comfort, it further suppressed my real spirit. Sixty percent of me remained in limbo all through my drinking days, until one day the alcohol no longer provided the relief I craved. I knew I needed help.

The reconnection with my spirit did not happen all at once, like turning on a switch. It was a more gradual process. I have noticed that some people really aren't ready to let go of their secrets and therefore prolong the process. They are hanging on for dear life because they feel that if they let go, they'll lose their identity. Or they may have not really forgiven themselves yet; in some way they still feel responsible. They keep restimulating all the past abuse and the issues around it because they still think they should have done something differently. In their resistance to letting go, they turn up the volume on the tape of accusations that runs in their head: "I shouldn't have told. I feel guilty because I didn't. I could have done otherwise."

If people balk at becoming reconnected and moving forward, they still need to work on forgiving themselves. The seven days of forgiveness activities may need to be extended. You will know when you have truly forgiven yourself because you will no longer struggle with those feelings of guilt and regret; you will feel a lot of energy around the idea of moving forward.

Eventually, as people become reassociated with their spirit, the energy once attached to the secret becomes focused on this fascinating new life they have and how they are now able to make real connections with other people. They feel flashes of power and confidence that keep them moving forward when their minds become murky with doubt. Like the sun's rays that gradually take precedence over the lights of the city, at a certain point there will be all this energy around who they really are and very little around the past. It will fade like the night.

I Would Rather Be an Interesting Person Than a Person with an Interesting Past

Vestiges of my victim identity remain in me today. My victim behavior has a particular way of emerging when I am in a personal crisis. I can observe it every time I walk away from a conflict in a close relationship instead of staying to work it out. Like shame, this fear in me is like tar. It clings to me and I have to scrape it off. It takes a long time before we stop thinking like a victim, but we can stop *acting* like a victim *today*—right now.

It's said that when you first enter the process of recovery, you have a spiritual awakening. Then about a year later you have a *rude* awakening: You realize that you have to look beyond the past sources of your problem and start making some changes in the present. Recovery is the courage to observe your behavior as objectively as an honest auto mechanic looking under the hood to evaluate what's working and what's not. People get stuck at this point because they have spent a lifetime looking back in time for the cause of their problems.

However, we need to stop hiding behind our secrets and defining ourselves in terms of them. People who go around calling themselves "survivors" are actually defining themselves in terms of their traumas. "Victim" becomes their identity. Some may say, "Well, at least it's something." Believe me, it's poisonous to our spirit. Being a victim is no identity for a healthy person, and being a survivor is not enough either. We have to thrive!

What Do You Value?

The key to defining your spirit is not through what happened to you in life but what you value. I would say that nearly all our values are conscious decisions based on what we have been exposed to in our experience of life. You need to look at each value you have chosen over the years and decide which ones you want to discard or add or elevate or demote in value. The goal in recovery is to value yourself above all else.

In the task of defining your spirit, you need to explore all your old inherent values and make a conscious decision about how important they are in your life now. By examining them you can clarify what's really important. For instance, I place a high value on family relationships because my family did. Every Sunday, my relatives would come from the neighborhood and other sections of Brooklyn, each bringing a cake or a dish to a daylong family get-together. However, the value I placed on family relationships became confused with the value they placed on food. Mom always said it was so important because of the Depression. Because her generation sometimes went hungry when they were growing up, food was really a big deal later on when they could afford it. We had porterhouse steaks and lamb chops. When I went to the local butcher shop to buy meat for the family, I felt very important. Other families might eat bologna on their sandwiches, but my mom always had me buy ham and roast beef. It appeared that we really loved each other because we spent extra money on the food we ate together.

Today, the value I place on food has remarkably diminished. This change is what melted the pounds away, not focusing on weight loss. Food is no longer connected with intimacy, it's not how I say "I love you." I value food for just what it is, delicious nourishment for the body, not for the spirit. I do not eat it to seek intimacy. I want that from real-life people. I don't eat to relieve pain because I am connected with people who will nourish me when I am in pain. My relationship to other kindred spirits and to their energy is now the driving force in life, not my connection to food.

That doesn't mean I don't enjoy food, and I still love certain favorites, like cheese. There's nothing wrong with liking to eat, and in fact, it would be crazy not to enjoy food. However, it is no longer the highlight of my day. Now food is just food. The intensity is gone, like an old flame who no longer makes your heart skip a beat but returns to being just another person. My life is so abundant and so full and there are so many more important things to be focused on that eating has become just another part of the day. Now food is seasoned with conversation and consumed among the energy of kindred spirits. It is an interesting side dish rather than the main course of my life.

As I examined my list of values and how they had changed over the years, I found that a new one had been added along the way: integrity. I love the word. I used to think it was for dignitaries, and I would never have believed that I would say it about myself, but *I have integrity*. To me, it is simply that I know I'm not going to compromise what I value. I can't *not* be true to myself. My masks have fallen apart and been discarded. I am Janet—loving, caring, abundant, giving.

Find Someone Who Believes in You

Once you have a well-defined identity, you are ready to relate to the world, but after being isolated for so long, it's going to be a little scary. You need to find someone who will encourage and nurture you, someone who will believe in you, especially during those doubtful moments when you find it hard to believe in yourself.

When I was finally ready to reconnect with others, I had the great fortune of finding someone who believed in me. Marie was not the usual mentor or role model most people describe; she hadn't done anything spectacular with her own life. She was so important to me because she believed in me. She had an unshakable, blind faith in my potential at a time when I didn't have a clue. Marie urged me to go back to college and become a therapist. Her belief in me helped me to go ahead and do what I wanted to with my life. I will always be thankful for her.

Many people who have been battered or abused have been given a lifetime of negative messages. You may not have had someone who believed in you, who looked you in the eye and said you were important, who gave you the message that you could accomplish whatever you set out to accomplish. You can't do anything about the past, but you can find people now who will believe in you. They may make all the difference.

Finding Nurturers

When you are around people, even those you know well, pay attention to how they make you feel. Be conscious of the way you respond to what they say and especially what they convey to you not with words but merely by their presence. One of my problems in early recovery was my lack of balance in selecting people to be close to: I forgot to get as well as give. I spent all of my energy trying to be there for others, but I never got anything in return. Those of us who do for others have to be cautious about balancing the amount of time we spend giving and how much time we spend getting back. There has to be proportion. We have to think of ourselves. This is not being selfish; we need to take care of ourselves, because if we're not getting what we need, we're eventually going to be unable to be there for anyone else.

I am not telling you to cut people out of your life (unless they're actually harmful to you), but be aware of how certain individuals affect you. For instance, when conversation starts to feel like work, you're around an energy sapper. There are people you may be fond of, who may even be wonderful, but who wear you out at the end of each visit. You feel as if you've been in a battle even though you didn't have a fight. In fact, nothing negative may have happened, but they leave you feeling depleted. Sometimes it's because they're wonderful people stuck in a fear-based persona, or they could just be apathetic. Nevertheless, they sap your energy, and when you need nurturing, you will be wise to be aware of your time spent with them. If you are feeling down or confused, it's good to be around people who act healthier than you feel at the present moment. Healthy people are energy boosters.

You need to become conscious of what you need and who you can get it from. Everyone needs comforting and love; everyone needs to be taken care of sometimes. You deserve to be nurtured by people who care. Let them into your life.

Mentors

If you didn't get what you needed from your parents, you may benefit from finding a mentor. A mentor is someone who possesses qualities you admire and want to emulate and who will help you become all you want to be.

Mentors tell you the truth about yourself in a friendly way. They have no hooks in you, no ulterior motives, no dreams to live through you, no wish to control you. They are successful at what you want to do and are willing to coach you. You can learn from mentors just by being around them, meeting their friends, seeing how they interact with people, and listening to their opinions.

If you can't find a personal mentor, you can study people who are doing what you want to do. You can read autobiographies of people who have something you desire for yourself and study the way they live. I always wanted to be a great speaker, full of charisma, and an excellent presenter. I didn't personally know any great speakers, so I started studying people's speeches or the way a person grabbed a small group's attention at a party. I discovered that the best presenters simply told interesting stories. I started doing that, too. I'm not there yet, but I get better and better. Simply by observing people I admire I have moved that much closer to being who I want to be.

Identifying your spirit, examining your values, and making changes in your life does take some work, but if you take those first steps, you will find that the Real You will emerge, blossom, and flourish. You owe it to yourself and everyone around you to be the best you can be, and this can only happen if you take care of your needs. Go ahead—you deserve it!

ACTIVITIES
Days 38-50

Day 38: The Affirmation to Thrive

Read this affirmation tonight and for the next fifteen nights before going to bed and any other time when you may feel yourself slipping back into victim thinking.

A victim is a prisoner of fear, shame, and rage

A survivor has alchemized these feelings into forgiveness.

A victim can't forget.

A survivor has remembered.

A victim suffers much but feels nothing.

A survivor feels everything and can laugh.

A victim keeps a "dirty little secret."

A survivor has washed clean in the salt of truth.

A victim's life is a heavy burden.

A survivor travels light to a further vision.

A victim is chained to the past and fears the future.

A survivor is here, today, and free.

A victim hopes to survive.

A survivor works to thrive.

We are the strongest people alive.

Day 39: Who Else Can You Be?

It is the intention of this book to help people change their perceptions of themselves. You may be convinced that you are the way you are and will always be that way, but that's why you're stuck! As deeply as you may believe that your perception can't be changed, I believe it can. I can show you how.

The famous perceptual puzzle shown opposite has always been very telling for me as a therapist. If you look at the picture you may see one of two things: a beautiful young woman or a very old woman. What is so interesting to me is that some people can only see the lines that make up the face of the old woman or only the lines of the young woman, but they can't see both. Sometimes they become upset and even angry if they can't see both. "How could something be there and I can't see it?" they ask heatedly.

If you can't see both women, you may be limiting your vision of who you are and your perception of possibilities. The harder you try to see the alternative perception, the more you may be struggling with your single image view and your persistence in believing there are no options.

If you can't see both women right away, don't despair. Maybe you will have to walk away and come back to the picture another time or look at it backward in a mirror.

This diagnostic exercise shows how perceptions are not rock solid but can be changed. This news may overwhelm you and even shake your belief in yourself. Allow yourself time to absorb the fact that change is possible and be encouraged by this. You can open yourself up to a whole new world of possibilities. Open your eyes and your mind and you will eventually see both women in the picture and so much more!

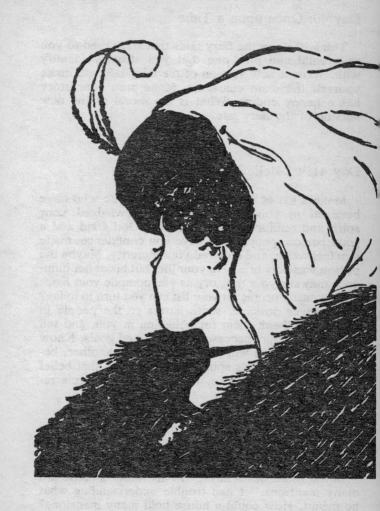

Day 40: Once upon a Time

Think back on the fairy tales that were read to you as a child and pick one that you strongly identify with. Write a new version of the fairy tale and make yourself the main character. Make sure your story has a happy ending. What is the moral of the new version of the fairy tale?

Day 41: "I Believe in You"

Make a list of all the people in your life who have believed in you—people who acknowledged your spirit and reinforced that you were God's kid and a good person, people who gave you confidence, made you feel warm, and honored your integrity. Maybe the person was only briefly in your life, but his or her influence may stir your memory as you compile your list.

How many people on your list can you turn to today?

Wherever possible, write letters to the people in your past, thank them for believing in you, and tell them about your successes, failures, and goals. Know that one day you will play that role for another, believing in someone's spirit at a time when that belief makes all the difference. In that way, the circle remains unbroken.

Day 42: Abundance for All

In the Bible, Jesus says, "In my father's house are many mansions." I had trouble understanding what he meant. How could a house hold many mansions?

Then one day I connected this mysterious Bible verse to my new value of abundance. What I had once considered abundant was a mere fraction of what was really possible. The potential for abundance is so much greater than we think.

This is especially true of emotional abundance. Believe me, there is more than enough love to go around. People who have been deprived of their emotional needs develop a perception of a world of scarcity, where there is never enough to go around. This exercise is designed to expand your perception of emotional abundance and reframe that perception of emotional scarcity.

At the top of a piece of paper, write "Abundance for All." Divide the paper into three columns. Label the column on the left "What I Need"; the middle column, "How to Get It"; and the column on the right, "Effect on Others." For each thing you list in your "needs" column, write concrete ways in which you can go about getting it in the middle column. Then take a few moments to consider how fulfilling this need will affect those you are close to, both positively and negatively.

For example, you may need more leisure time. In order for this to be achieved, you may have to work less hours or drop some of your activities outside the home. This may mean a reduced income. Would having less money be a hardship to your loved ones? Or would spending more leisure time with them have a positive effect? Other needs might be time alone, a new career, more education, or a change in a relationship. Ask yourself now what you need the most.

When you have finished with your list, review it and decide which need can be the most readily achieved. Make it your number one priority. Then study the right-hand column for a while and see what it tells you about emotional scarcity. Is giving to yourself really going to result in others getting less? You may be surprised at the answer.

Day 43: The Nurturing Parent

Write on a sheet of paper what you would like your ideal nurturing parent to say to you, for example, "I love you," "You're beautiful," "I like you just the way you are," "I'm so proud of you."

Using your left hand (or your right hand if you are left-handed), write the sentences again.

Stand up and read aloud the words you would like to hear from your ideal nurturing parent. Read them in the way you would like to hear them—warmly, lovingly, slowly, and tenderly.

In your journal, describe how this activity made you feel.

Day 44: Nurturing the Spirit—A Guided Imagery

Prepare for this exercise by doing some deep breathing. Lie comfortably and close your eyes. Imagine your spirit as a young plant that has been nearly killed off living unattended in a dark place. Notice how pale its leaves are and how they droop. Notice how thirsty the plant is and how the soil is depleted and dry as dust. Take the plant out of the dark place to nourish it. Find a bigger pot to put it in and fill it up with fresh, rich soil full of good nutrients. Wash the dust off the leaves and give the plant a careful watering—not too much and not too little, just enough to soak the roots well. Put your plant in a sunny window and watch it grow. Pretty soon tiny new green leaves begin to sprout on the branches, and you can all but hear the roots burrowing deeper into the nutrient-rich soil.

Your spirit may be like that neglected plant. No one has cared for it, even though it doesn't require more than a few minutes of your attention every day. Can you care for your spirit that much today? Ask it what it needs and give it what you can. You may be astonished to see how quickly it will respond to even a little nurturing with vigorous new growth.

Day 45: Nurturing Yourself—A Guided Visualization

Sit comfortably, close your eyes, and relax. Breathe in and out ten times, focusing on your breathing. In your imagination you are walking along the beach. What do you see, feel, hear, and smell? Now sit down on the sand. Feel the water as it comes onto shore and watch it go back out.

There is a gift here for you. You need to start digging in the sand until the gift appears. When you have found your gift, look it over, touch it, listen to it, and smell it. Put the gift in a safe place where you can enjoy it whenever you want to remember this special moment to nurture yourself.

Day 46: Three People You Admire

Describe three people, famous or not famous, whom you admire. They must already have something you want. Describe what it is about them that you identify with so strongly. Describe how you are like them.

Day 47: Mentor Me

Make a list of all the people you know in your field of endeavor who have the knowledge you need and who might be willing to give their time to guide you. Sometimes the best mentors are those who do not possess the self-centered, driven nature needed for success. They have the talent, they love to keep it honed, and they are likely to have more time. However, do not assume that because a person is successful that he or she is too busy to respond to a request from you for information, resources, recommendations of people to study with, or whatever it is you need. Often the mentor is very busy but has reached a point where he or she wants to give back.

One of the problems we addicts share is making blanket judgments about whole groups of people and staying in the dark by refusing to give ourselves what we need. It amazes me how many people in recovery go muddling along without a mentor. It just never occurs to them to find one. We all deserve them, however, for their wisdom and experience prevent us from making expensive, time-wasting mistakes. The beauty of mentors is they can serve as positive role models and guide us toward our goals by pointing out both our strengths and our weaknesses.

Go over your list of potential mentors. Have you forgotten anyone? Select one name, and by the end of the week, make contact by telephone or letter.

Day 48: What Are You Doing for Yourself These Days?

Read through the daily entries in your journal describing what you have done for yourself each day. Summarize your progress. Has your ability to care for yourself increased? How about the quality of care? Describe any resistance to taking care of yourself that you may be going through. Have others begun to notice the fact that you're taking better care of yourself these days? How do they react and how do you respond to their reactions?

Day 49: What You Value

The 10 percent of you that is physical values a home, food, and creature comforts. The 30 percent of you that is your thinking, feeling self values knowledge, variety, acceptance, peace of mind, and other emotional values. However, the value words of the 10 and the 30 percent are not energy words and therefore cannot describe your spirit, the 60 percent of you that can't be seen, felt, or touched.

The purpose of this activity is to invoke your spirit by naming its qualities, using words that truly resonate in you when you say them, words full of good energy.

The following list of words are full of that good

energy. Say them out loud, each word preceded by "I am." Pay attention to the words that resonate the strongest.

Abundant	Sensuous	Humorous
Sensual	Loving	Caring
Nurturing	Free spirited	Exciting
Spontaneous	Creative	Passionate
Radiant	Translucent	Powerful
Enthusiastic	Compassionate	Freedom loving
Expressive	Vigorous	Sunny
Illuminating	Invigorating	Comforting
Warmhearted	Amorous	Cherishable
Endearing	Fascinating	Wonderful
Lovable	Heroic	Mysterious
Courageous	Incandescent	Encouraging
Mirthful	Generous	Delightful
Exhilarating	Scintillating	Fruitful
Interesting	Energetic	Merry
Plentiful	Luminous	Dynamic
Curious	Exuberant	Vivacious
Persistent	Ambitious	Playful
Robust	Expansive	Attractive
Stimulating	Desirable	Cheerful
High reaching	Animated	Carefree
Adventurous	Light-hearted	
Joyful	Buoyant	
Vital	Enchanting	
Inspiring	Captivating	ALIVE

Which energy words evoked the strongest emotional response in you? These are your values, for they best describe your spirit. Say them to yourself as your new "I am" affirmation daily for the remainder of the ninety days.

Day 50: Reassociating—A Visual Sculpture

This activity is especially healing for those who have gone through childhood trauma. It is a resculpturing by guided imagery of that child's spirit before the dissociation. The goal is to reassociate that spirit through images. Prepare for this activity with a deep breathing or other relaxation exercise. Play some music that makes you feel serene and peaceful. Lie comfortably and close your eyes.

Search your mind for the little child who was so full of life and free of spirit before the onset of the harmful messages. When that child is clearly in mind, take its face lovingly in your hands and feel the child's silken skin and the delicate contours of its little head. Feel the vibrancy of that being and the eagerness to experience life in all its mysteries.

Now, implore that impatient child to sit for a moment while you take a lump of modeling clay and sculpt the child's head. You are an experienced mental sculptor. The contours of the face are beautiful under your fingertips. The child's spirit still vibrates there. Keeping your eyes closed, place your hands gently on the contours of your face and trace the child's spirit that still lives in your being. Now return to your sculpture and slowly, gently adjust the features to become your own. Tell your spirit that you are now one.

VI

Finding
Your Heart

The famous psychiatrist Fritz Perls says there are three questions that puzzle everyone: who we are, where we come from, and where we are going. These three questions are at the core of our concern as human beings. We have already determined who we are by identifying our values. In the process, we have examined where we came from and have retained whatever it is that we still value from the past. Only at this point are we equipped to explore our destiny.

I really believe you have to have a strong identity before you can find your purpose. If your identity is still shattered, the energy dissipates. If you are still living in the uncomfortable disguise of a false identity, your purpose is bound to be off course, for it will be twisted. How can you determine your purpose in life when you don't really know who you are?

I like to tell the story about the retired man and his wife who were driving down the highway, speeding like mad. He turned to his wife and said, "I don't know where we're going, but we're making terrific time." I think this story describes many people who are moving fast but really don't have any direction.

It seems that the hardest thing you ever have to figure out is what you really want to do with your life. I believe it's such an incredibly difficult task because it shakes the foundations of a shame-based person, radically shifting the focus from the past to the future. Nevertheless, just as no other person in the world can tell you what your values are, you yourself must find your own meaning or you will end up at someone else's destination.

As you think about your vision, don't consider the obstacles, whether you're good enough, or whether you deserve it. Our minds are accustomed to talking us out of what we really want to protect us from the disappointment of failure. If I had sat down years ago and realistically tried to plan how I could afford to fulfill my dream of going to college, I never would have gone. However, I believe the mind tries to figure a way around obstacles once it has a vision motivated by our deepest desires.

What's Your Mission?

Have you ever watched a weed come out of the ground? It's very aggressive. The soil above it gets disturbed, but the plant doesn't care. It knows what it wants. It wants the sunlight, and it will go to great lengths to get it. Its mission is to grow and nothing can get in its way, not even a slab of concrete!

When people in recovery finally start doing what

they're here to do, everybody had better step aside. They have all this wonderful excitement and energy, and they have been idling so long that once they get moving they're like children in their determination. They want to make things happen, not out of fear but out of desire, and that makes all the difference.

When kids want something like, say, a candy bar, they'll ask you for it twenty times an hour until you give them the candy to shut them up! They are relentless, and they are unafraid to let people know they want something and they want it badly. If they don't get what they want, they don't take it personally either. They just plan their next ambush. They don't feel the rejection because they haven't been affected yet by all the negative messages that tell us something is wrong with us if we don't get what we want. We should take a lesson from the children.

Everyone has a mission, not necessarily a calling or a profession, but a reason for being. It might be motherhood or learning everything you can about a subject that interests you. I know someone whose mission is to see every major city on the globe. He's up to eight and says he has fourteen to go. He works hard, saves his money for travel, and enjoys looking forward to his adventures as much as talking about the ones he's already had. His vision of the world is fascinating to me, for it is fascinating to him and his passion is contagious.

The real difficulty lies not in fulfilling your mission, but finding it. We are so accustomed to devaluing ourselves that we also devalue our mission, whatever that may be. A mission in life comes directly out of a person's values. If you are unsure about yours, read over your list of values from Day Forty-nine (page 176) as well as your daily "I am" affirmations. Because values are energy words, they empower your mission as well as help define it. As you look over your energy words, what kind of activity comes to mind?

I know that my mission is to make a difference in the lives of others, and everything I do is in pursuit of that mission, with all my energy and focus undistracted by anything that would deter me. At one point in my life, I consciously held myself back and didn't speak up when I had an opinion because I was afraid I wouldn't be accepted. That fear, not my mission, was the driving force in my life.

Once you have a solid identity, you will no longer be stuck in the fear. You will be too busy following your mission to give it more than a passing thought. In the meantime, the fear will be there, and it's honest to admit to having it. The goal is not to banish fear but to act in spite of it. You have two choices in those instances: fear with action or fear without action. Once your action is empowered by your values, your fear will melt away.

When you have a mission, the power you tap into will be so great that others will begin to respond to you differently. They will experience you as being purposeful, yet comfortable to be around because of your clarity of purpose. Best of all, you will feel comfortable, for your confusion will be gone; grounded in a solid self-identity, your mission will lead you, empower you, and fulfill you.

When I Found My Heart

Life has moments that are unforgettable, and part of my driving force is made up of those moments. I have always wanted to help people like myself, but if I hadn't had an experience out in the Arizona desert several years ago, I'm not sure I would be so convinced that I'm on the right journey. As the years go by, this wonderful experience becomes like an epiphany, because its impact was so powerful.

My struggle for a spiritual life had taken me many places, including a Native American retreat in the foothills of the Arizona desert. I'm from Brooklyn, and I don't have a real connection to nature due to the massive city blocks where I grew up. I felt out of my realm in nature, but I went to the retreat because I wanted to explore the new me and relate to others. I knew very little of the Native American's spiritual quest and came to the retreat not knowing what to expect.

We were asked to go into the mountains and find something that might be symbolic of who we were. I always had difficulty with these artsy-craftsy assignments. I couldn't think of what I could find with all this nature around. Eventually I thought about the rose and the heart. They were meaningful to me since childhood as symbols of Saint Theresa. I knew it would be impossible to find a rose in the desert, and as for finding a heart, I couldn't imagine what form it could take—maybe a pebble, a rock, or a twig in the shape of a heart.

From a distance, the landscape looked like the one I had seen in many cowboy movies, but actually walking through those foothills was something brand-new. As I made the gradual climb, the shadow of the mountains looming above me, for the first time I became aware of the true meaning of the word *desolate*. I mean, there was nothing, *nada!* I realized the place was so beautiful *because* it was desolate. It was also mystical. The mountains and rocks that jutted straight out of the earth were like ancient forms that spelled out some secret meaning. Would they help me find what I was looking for? Suddenly, something caught my eye. Right at my feet, wedged in the dirt, I found a gold heart-shaped pin. I couldn't believe it. How could this happen? I asked myself. We're miles from anywhere. What does it all mean?

I was overwhelmed. The likelihood of the tiny pin being discovered at my feet was just too much to take in. I kept trying to analyze what happened. I believe God steered me toward that heart because I wanted it.

All my life, my dilemma had been trying to understand the spiritual—something I couldn't see, hear, feel, or touch. I never really understood God and probably never will, but now I trust Him. When I found that heart-shaped pin, I felt connected to the great Spirit, a healing force of goodness in the universe that is outside of myself. I interpreted finding my heart as God's way of telling me that no matter what I want, I should take the action to get it. I would get what I wanted, and if it wasn't right for me, God would stop me dead in my tracks.

Finding my heart is about the connection with my spirit and my connection with God. It is my own personal trinity. Until I found the heart in the mountains, I had a difficult time understanding what spirituality is. The analytical, rational part of me that based everything on what can be seen, felt, or touched kept me from being connected. Once I let go, I was connected. That's what let go and let God means to me today.

When I was disconnected from my internal spirit and from the external spirit, I existed in a twilight state of perpetual dis-ease. Now I radiate. Once you have the power of your spirit connecting with the spiritual, you plug into an enormous force. Since that day in Arizona, I know in my heart that I am God's kid and that He will help me get everything I need. That connection now empowers my life, and I am free of worry because I know I am not alone.

The Paradoxes of Recovery: Becoming Contrary

Recovery is full of paradoxes that make the process one of many surprises. The paradox of letting go in order to be connected was only the first I experienced. In recovery, each symptom of the disease is turned around, and the remedy is found in its polar opposite. Recovery means making a turnaround from apathy to empathy, from rigidity to creativity, from sadness to humor, from reactive to proactive, and from responsible to responsive. Recovery is being turned right side out and inside in.

From Apathy to Empathy

I think the worst thing about depression is how it flattens the ability to experience joy. I know people who actually lose their sense of smell when they are deeply depressed and are only made aware of their loss when they step into an elevator one day and suddenly take in the mingled aromas of cigarette smoke and perfume.

The terrible part about depression is it makes nothing worthwhile enough to expend effort to achieve. Apathetics are depressed from repressing their spirit, an action that consumes so much of their energy that they don't have enough left to go out and live. You almost get the sense that they're asleep.

For some of us, recovery means tempering our empathy. Caring and doing too much for others is just as harmful, especially when we're motivated by fear of not being liked. That doesn't help anyone either. Empathy is a gift to the world, but empathy overdone burns us out and immobilizes us just as apathy does. In recovery we learn to give from a healthy core being, not out of sickness or as an effort to get someone to like us. We learn to see empathy as being connected to others in a meaningful way and not just another way to keep doing for others.

From Rigidity to Creativity

Rigidity is a negative state in which creativity cannot flourish. Disconnected people become adept at denying their negativity, but this denial consumes all their energy, leaving their ability for creative expression limited. I believe this is the reason so many artists chemically alter their minds with alcohol or drugs; they are trying to create an artificial positive mental environment in order to produce.

We all start out creative. Pay a visit to any kindergarten class and you will notice that creativity being expressed with great exuberance by one and all. Inside all of us lies a store of unexpressed creativity, filled to overflowing. It has remained suppressed for a long time, but it can't find an outlet in a state of rigidity.

Rigidity is one of the most commonly observed characteristics of disconnected people. Control freaks are an obvious example, but we are all afraid to take a chance or express our uniqueness because we can't risk making a mistake. Disconnected people also have a hard time exploring alternatives or seeing other options. If you had difficulty seeing the second woman in the activity for Day Thirty-nine (page 169), you may have a problem with rigidity.

How does someone who has been disconnected for a long time break out of that rigidity? The answer is, a little at a time. Think of your mind as you would your body: If a part of it had been bound up in one position for a long time, the muscles would be weak and would need special exercise. A rigid mind is the same. It's not ready to create with the exuberance of a child, using bold strokes and strong colors. It feels too uncomfortable.

Rather than think of creativity as something artists do, I like to think of it as an aesthetic that is present even in the most ordinary things. It is an attitude that can be developed toward everything we touch in an everyday way.

The message of Saint Theresa is that she did the ordinary in extraordinary ways. If you are unsure about following your creative urges, begin with a "touch of the practical," like straightening your closets and drawers. Don't wait, as I used to, until it seems like a heavy chore and feels intolerable. Now I do the job a little at a time. I keep the everyday things in my life somewhat organized—my desk, my makeup tray—because I have found that it organizes my thoughts to organize the small things I touch every day.

Being spontaneous is another form of creativity. It's really the opposite of rigidity. Some people are terrified of impulsive behavior. If you said to them, "Let's take a drive tonight. There's a full moon," they would go into a panic and give a dozen reasons why they couldn't. I've learned to let go of the dozen reasons for a moment to consider that moon rising over the mountains. Spontaneity can also be as simple as driving home a different way, noticing people, flowers, houses.

Let your creativity resurface a little at a time. Let even the smallest things in your everyday life be an outlet for expression. You will soon find that imagination and beauty will constantly flow from you.

From Tragedy to Comedy

There are times when I feel overwhelmed by how many tragic things have happened to people, but I don't allow myself to focus on it for long. How long can you really listen to unanswerable questions like "Why me?"

People who continually bring up their tragic history become like Joe #@*%!, the character in the "Li'l Abner" comic strip with an unprintable last name. There was a permanent rainstorm over Joe's head, and he was always under an umbrella. People were not happy to see him coming. However, I have found that the funniest people I know have had a lot of tragedy in their lives. Take Richard Pryor. One of the reasons he's so unique is he can make fun of himself. I have noticed I always get the biggest laughs when I tell a story about myself in a vulnerable moment.

People who have been abused and have played the victim role for a long time have to cultivate humor. They have spent a lifetime without laughter because they have been stuck in the mire of depression and self-loathing. Their spirits have been unable to see joy in anything for so long that they have trouble recognizing the comic element inherent in so much of life. Along the process of recovery, however, these same long-faced people begin to experience a little fun, and when their spirit gets fully activated, they become like kids who just discovered a store where all the candy is free.

If you are unable to laugh right now, don't despair. It will come a little at a time, and soon you'll be able to laugh at yourself, and that's the best kind of laughter there is. People in early recovery need to remember not to take themselves so seriously. Learning to cultivate laughter may seem like a frivolous assignment, but I mean it in dead earnest. A lightness of being does not in any way minimize our stories. Our story will always be with us. However, to be able to find humor in our lives will help us move beyond our traumas to full, productive futures full of laughter, joy, and smiles.

From Reactive to Proactive

Some people are reacting constantly, always waiting for something to happen. They're in a state of perpetual unpredictability. Actually, there is a logic to their reactive state: By simply letting things happen to them, they only have to put out just enough energy to get by. Reactive people, however, can get stuck for years, always waiting, never going after what they want.

Becoming proactive means planning ahead. It is strategizing to figure out ways to get what you desire rather than waiting until something happens that you can react to. If you were playing football, it would mean switching to offense from defense. Every Sunday night, no matter where I am—at home or in a hotel room—I take out my calendar and figure out my entire week. I plan out who I want to have dinner with and how I will spend my evenings. I figure out my work priorities, I make lists of people to call. Guess what? I never find myself roaming alone through a bookstore feeling empty. I don't wait to let life happen to me, and unless I plan to be alone, I'm not alone. I'm proactive in everything I do. I love my life. I make it happen.

From Responsible to Responsive

I have noticed that whenever I talk to patients at "Your Life Matters" about responsibility I get a negative reaction. I believe *responsibility* is an especially problematic word for addicts. Being overly conscientious is one of the first defenses children who have been abused employ; it is a way for them to compensate for their self-loathing and lack of identity. They are so shame based that they often take on more responsibility than they can handle just so they can feel good about themselves. I used to feel responsible for taking care of everyone. It was so much work, and no matter how much I did, I never felt as if it was enough.

Responsibility in its true sense has nothing to do with taking care of others. It's about our ability to respond. Remember how you responded to the world when you were a child, before all the negative messages? That's responsibility.

Our actions should have nothing to do with unnecessarily assumed responsibility. My *reactions* to things tend to come from the past, a kind of knee-jerk feeling that something must be done and I'd better do it. However, I have learned to *respond*—I can feel and acknowledge—and do something or nothing at all. My actions are up to me—I make conscious decisions and smart choices, doing what's best for me and everyone involved.

When I reframe *responsibility* to "response—ability" or the ability to respond, my patients feel good just thinking about it. It's no longer an obligation, but a positive attribute. It's taking control of yourself and choosing how you behave.

Similarly, I redefine maturity as "emotional maturity." It's a wonderful gift: the body's capacity to experience life through communication with others. People who have this grown-up approach to their feelings don't drag you down. When unexpected things happen, they're cool about it and don't take the matter so personally, as if everything revolved around them. They don't react without thinking; instead, they experience life and respond to it.

From reactive to proactive, from responsible to responsive—you may wonder how all these radical changes can possibly come about when you have spent a lifetime failing at life or losing weight. Exactly how these changes happen requires a leap of faith; you must trust yourself. As a result of taking action, you will be exploring who you are and why you are here, and you will find yourself giving up harmful, long-held beliefs that are holding you back. You will become reconnected to your spirit and experience an abundance beyond your wildest dreams.

Eventually your life will spring forward, and your former existence of scarcity and isolation will be a dim memory. There will be so much more to the world than you ever imagined that you will find yourself waking up each day vibrating with energy, eager to do the best you can and to enjoy as much of the abundance of life as possible.

ACTIVITIES
Days 51-74

Day 51: Invoking the Spirit

The purpose of this activity is to invoke the spirit, to bring it forth by calling it by name. You may not, however, have a name yet for what or who this spirit is. Instead, you will use the power of images.

Assemble a collage of the Real You from magazines, photographs, paintings, or other visual sources. Depict your spirit in all its joyfulness before the imprint of the negative messages. Look for metaphors, images (not necessarily people) that are meaningful to your spirit. It might be a waterfall or an eagle. Without using words, select images of this pure being who experiences life with such zest. In the process, you will create images of how you want the world to experience you.

Day 52: What's Your Mission as Expressed by the Child?

In your journal, write about the future you envisioned for yourself when you were a child. What did you want to be? When did you first start thinking about your ambitions? Explore those options you chose as a child, not to consider a career change but for the values inherent in those choices.

The child who wants to be a fire fighter values courage and service. The astronaut values adventure and scientific exploration. The nurse values helping people. The movie star values fame and glamour.

Day 53: What's Your Mission? Your Most Exciting Moment?

Prepare for this activity by deep breathing or progressive relaxation exercises. Lie comfortably and let your mind become like a darkened room with a large movie screen. Project onto that screen an exciting moment in your life. What is the source of the excitement? Are you alone or with other people? Were you an observer or a participant? How old were you? How did the excitement make you feel? Where exactly did you experience it? In the heart? The head? The body? Were there any consequences to the excitement? How could you re-create this excitement in a way that would be beneficial to yourself and others?

Here is an example of what this activity can reveal: For years, one of my patients had felt stuck in her job, which consisted of crunching numbers. While doing this exercise, she saw a scene flash in her mind that completely surprised her. She had been working on a local election, and their candidate won. As she made her way to the clubhouse for the postelection celebration, she could hear the revelry a block away, and her heart filled with an enormous joy. She never felt so happy. After doing the visualization, she realized with a rush of excitement that she needs to be involved with people and a cause they shared. Although she didn't run right out and join a group, within the year she was involved in an afterschool program teaching math and accounting to students who couldn't afford a tutor. I wasn't at all surprised to find that she had also helped form a group with students and parents to convince the local school board to fund a regular tutorial program. Now she's working at the program part-time and is busier than ever, but her stores of energy have increased far more than what she has taken on. Her eyes glow when she tells you about the student she tutored who just won a college scholarship. She has found her mission.

Day 54: What's Your Mission? Interim Goals

Many people feel guilty for doing what they want because for so long they never felt worthy enough to respond to their own needs. They conditioned themselves to always do for others and felt selfish if they thought about themselves. But forcing ourselves to do things we don't want but feel obliged to do undermines our creativity. Fortunately, the life force is as persistent as a child. If you begin this self-inquiry, what you really want to do rather than what you think you should be doing will become clear:

1. If you could achieve one thing in this world, what would it be?
2. What is one thing you can do *today* that would be a step toward achieving that goal?
3. Write your goal on a piece of paper, put it in your wallet, and carry it with you. Although a long-term, major goal will give you direction and purpose, smaller interim goals will stimulate and empower you. They might be learning a new skill, finishing a project, or financing a trip or a new car. After you do what must be done today, what would appeal to you to do with your free time?

Maybe something you enjoy but haven't done in a long time. Write down the activity and how you felt after making time for it.

4. Write down a goal you want to accomplish in six months. What do you want to accomplish in one year? Where do you want to be five years from now? Be specific. Put this list of goals in a safe place. Take it out and read it whenever your vision becomes clouded by doubt or an attack of shame.

Day 55: Tuning in to the Voice of Mission Control

The idea of having a mission determined by an outside force, whether beneficent or otherwise, is what bothers a lot of people about recovery. However, the reality is not about being controlled. Tuning in the voice of mission control is not about being controlled but controlling your mission, placing your hands on the wheel and moving forward.

Ask the following questions but do not answer them. Repeat the activity for the next seven days. Listen in prayer and meditation for a response:

What is it that I really enjoy? What gives me the greatest personal satisfaction? What special talent do I have that I contribute to the greater good in some small way? What can I take from that greater good and what can I give back of myself? Why am I here in this time and place and what have I been born to accomplish? What sign, what personal symbol that has meaning only to me, can I look for which will give me the answers I'm seeking?

Day 56: Spirit Meditation

Prior to meditating, read the following aloud several times. As you prepare for the meditation, visualize a universe connected by the energy of love.

> Spirit to Spirit
> Heart to Heart
> Connected through time and space
> by Grace
>
> Radiant, abundant light
> Sphere to Sphere
> Connected around and above
> with Love.

Day 57: "This Is My Little . . ."

I cringe every time I see a television commercial for a set of encyclopedias in which a mother is portrayed saying, "It would be nice to have a doctor in the family." Few people realize the negative influence of such a message—it threatens a child's ability to form his or her own identity. A parent's expectations can also be made known in many more subtle ways, but the effect is the same—a loss of opportunity to be the Real You. Some children are so spirited they resist this kind of manipulation by rejecting the profession desired for them by their parents out of rebellion. They make a *reactive* choice, not a *proactive* choice.

If the energy around forming your identity was distorted, the following is a *reframing* exercise in which the child in you can speak out. An example: In response to the parent's introduction, "This is my little ballerina,'' you might say, "Excuse me, it's true I like ballet dancing a lot, but I am not your little ballerina. I'm God's kid and right now my assignment is to be a kid and explore everything that's safe for me to explore. I don't know right now what I want to be, but here is what interests me a lot . . .''

List five things you were passionate about as a child.

Day 58: Finding Your Heart—Collage

Assemble a collage of pictures and small objects that gives a visual representation of your connection to a higher spirit. The collage should represent not how you worship this beneficent force in the universe, but how you feel about God and how you experience God as an energy source in your life. The visuals you choose may have a certain color, texture, fragrance, or line that to you emotionally evokes these feelings.

Day 59: Your Own TV Show

You have just been given a regular half-hour television show. What are you going to call it? What kind of show is it? How will it be described in the new TV listings? Being able to define your purpose in a few short words may take a while, but when you get it right, it will click and you will have gained further clarity about your purpose in life.

Day 60: Mask Making

For this activity, you will need a roll of plaster-impregnated gauze that doctors use to make casts and sculptors use for casting. You can find it in art and medical supply stores. You will also need a bowl of water to dip the strips in, petroleum jelly, a towel, and acrylic paint plus things to decorate the mask with, such as ribbons, feathers, sequins, jewels, or whatever trim can be glued on to your mask once it is dried.

Allow plenty of time for mask making. Approach it as a ritual. When mask making is done as a psychodrama, the experience is enormously bonding and brings up many feelings. It has a way of tapping into creative aspects of our lives in a transcendental way. People often describe having spiritual experiences while the mask is being created.

Find some soft and meditative music to play, such as "The Fairy Ring" by Mike Rowland or a favorite piece of classical music.

1. Secure hair away from the face. Apply petroleum jelly to face, use plenty around hairline, eyelashes, and chin.
2. Dip gauze strips in water and press each one gently between your fingers to activate the plaster.
3. Place the strips on the face, one layer at a time. Leave space for breathing through nostrils or mouth.
4. Leave the mask on to dry for approximately ten minutes.
5. Carefully remove the mask. Puncture small holes in the sides and thread a piece of cord through each hole and secure with a knot.
6. Let it set and dry some more. When it is completely dry, decorate your mask, keeping in mind

that you are creating your spirit and its connection with spirituality. It may represent an animal, a bird, or something symbolic. When you are finished, you will also have a life mask of who you are at this point in your recovery.

Day 61: Mask Dance

For some reason people who are ashamed of their bodies, especially those who have been sexually abused, find dancing while wearing a mask an amazingly liberating experience. Concealing the face has a way of allowing shame to leave the body. As a result, people say they truly feel the rhythm and grace of movement for the first time. The restrictive, tentative movements shame-based people tend to make do not allow for real expression. Through unrestricted dance, the spirit can reveal how it feels about God and revel in this connection with a higher spirit.

To do your mask dance, you need complete privacy and the freedom that brings. Second, you need to find the right dance music. Choose your theme song if it's joyous and uplifting.

Wear clothing that is neither provocative nor constricting. Tie on your mask and begin with some loosening up movements as the music begins. Then, as you did as a child, merge your body with the rhythm and the beat and become one with the music. Allow your spirit to take over and move you.

One incest survivor described her first mask dance with tears in her eyes. She explained that the greatest damage that had been done by her sexual abuse was to her divinity, the knowledge that she is God's kid.

Every time she tried to express herself through dance she felt "like a slut" and never knew why until she dealt with the incest. Behind the mask, she lost that identity with the abuse. She could have been anyone. The feeling of anonymity was what her body found so exhilarating. It freed her to allow her pure and playful spirit to leap into the picture. Once the spirit in you starts dancing, it will greatly expand and make more flexible and fluid the boundaries of who you think you are.

I have loved to dance since the days I was a tiny tot on the bartops. The part of me who dances is still that little kid, and I've taken her out into the world where she still dances with her fullest heart but in my protective care.

Day 62: Nourishing the 60 Percent— Becoming Contrary

Cross your arms. Now uncross them and recross them in the other direction. What does the unhabitual way you cross your arms feel like? Do you feel as if your bones don't quite fit right? Do you feel suddenly awkward? Deliberately cross your arms in the unaccustomed way five times during the course of the following day and each time say the following affirmation: "I am contrary. I am unhabitual. I am paradoxical. I am flexible. I willingly adapt. I am controversial. I surprise myself. I am making a turnaround. I love to change."

Day 63: Slings and Arrows

As you begin to make your paradoxical turn-arounds, you will probably upset some people who don't want you to change. Keep in mind that at first it will feel very strange to maintain your contrary behavior, and you may have to do some conscious "scripted" actions before your changes become habitual. It is especially difficult to maintain these changes in stressful situations when your emotions are in a storm and you can't think clearly.

The following visualization is designed to establish your newly defined boundaries the next time you are under stress.

The next time someone confronts you and wants to penetrate you with a message that violates your sense of self, instead of responding in the heat of emotion, which by now we all know is embarrassing and ineffectual, try this technique:

Imagine you are enclosed behind an invisible protective shield or a powerful energy field that cannot be penetrated. On the other side of this shield the person is saying things about you that hurt and anger you. Instead of responding, cup your chin in your hand or pinch your earlobe. The gesture is to remind you that all you have to do is listen. People have a tendency to defend themselves instead of listening, but remember, you are behind your invisible protective shield. There is no need for shame or rage, you can just listen.

As you listen, tell yourself that what the person is saying has to do with his or her own perceptions, not who you are. The same is true in reverse: What you choose to say or not say has everything to do with your own unique perception. Evaluate what is being said without shame or rage and then respond in a way that reflects your integrity. It may be that you choose to say nothing at all; you may have to delay your response as a form of strategy: Maybe you don't trust your ability to keep from flying into a rage at this point, maybe you are afraid apologies will come rushing out of your mouth, or maybe you won't be able to give a reasoned and balanced reply without all the usual emotion clouding your message. Whatever your response, it will come out of respect for your own sense of self rather than as a reaction to feeling attacked.

Day 64: Sending Your Tyrant on a Three-Week Vacation

When you start breaking out of old patterns, your internal voice that broadcasts the old negative messages will go on alert. That tyrant within you who fights to maintain the status quo will have a major fear attack. Right now you are too busy to focus on its problems; you can't let its negative messages distract you from your progress in recovery. Here is a visualization to use whenever you need some relief:

Sit back or stretch out on the floor in a relaxed position. Close your eyes and begin breathing in and out. Focus on your breath for ten deep breaths. Now listen for the voice of your inner tyrant—that destructive, critical, judgmental voice that lives as a freeloader in your head. What do you see, hear, smell, and feel as you take in that voice? Is the voice that of a man, a woman, or a monster? Describe your tyrant as accurately as you can. Is it smiling, frowning, or raging? Is it nagging, sneering, snorting, giving you dirty looks, pointing a finger at you, or giving you the old silent treatment? What the hell is it that your tyrant wants you to do so much that you don't want to do? Remember why you don't want to do that.

Now imagine you are picking up the telephone. Call the airlines and buy your inner tyrant a ticket for a three-week vacation on the next flight out. Choose a nice place. Drive your tyrant to the airport and say good-bye as that boring and bothersome creature walks down the runway and into the plane. Drive home free of your tyrant's constant criticism and guilt tripping. Open the windows of the car and let the breezes in. Close the windows, turn the radio on LOUD, and find a song you can sing. Shout above the music or sing the words if you like that you are a terrific person to take such good care of even this negative part of you. If you find that your tyrant returns home early, repeat the exercise as frequently as necessary until one day, in disgust and frustration, your tyrant packs its bags and vacates the premises.

Day 65: Nourishing the 60 Percent—An Assignment in Spontaneity

Yes, it's possible to plan to be spontaneous, even though that may sound like a contradiction. For those of us who need to break out of our rigidity, it is necessary to take a conscious action. The assignment is to do something playful and unplanned within the next forty-eight hours, preferably with another person. You might buy yourself a little gift, take in a movie on a weeknight, or call an old friend you haven't heard from in a while. After you've had your fun, write about it in your journal. What feelings came up for you when you made the leap into spontaneity? What was the reaction by the other person or persons? Were they willing or unwilling to do something spontaneous?

Day 66: Nourishing the 60 Percent—The Extraordinary in the Ordinary

I like to think that at "Your Life Matters" we do nothing so out of the ordinary therapeutically, but we do the ordinary in an extraordinary way—we do it with care and love. Care and love are the motivating factors behind this activity in which creativity is applied to the ordinary. Notice something in your everyday environment that needs straightening up. Maybe it's your shoes, jewelry, or makeup tray. Maybe it's your kitchen utensil or spice drawer, your tool chest, or your recycling basket. Approach your tidying up as an act of creativity, and while you do it, appreciate the beauty of the ordinary. Take time and don't rush through to get to something important; make this task important.

Be aware of the objects that come into your hands. Examine them, discard or give away what is no longer useful, and leave the job well done. Every day, as you appreciate this little straightening up job, it will give your mind a message that it absorbs on many levels: Creativity can be applied to everything, and in doing so you're doing another thing to take care of yourself.

Day 67: Wings—A Guided Imagery

This activity is for your spirit, which has felt constricted for so long. It needs to take a few practice soars in your mind to get back in shape after being in hiding all these years.

Lie or sit comfortably and close your eyes. Breathe deeply and focus on your breath for ten breaths. Then begin to notice that something is happening to your shoulder blades. You are sprouting wings! You walk over to a full-length mirror and turn around. There they are: big, beautiful wings, like the ones angels fly with, attached to your shoulders and back. Slowly begin to move your wings until you are able to float out of the room.

Now you are climbing a hill, flapping your wings, and barely touching the ground between flaps. You reach the top of the hill and look around. It is the perfect place for a takeoff. You flap and flap your wings with more and more strength until they begin to carry you upward and you are soaring effortlessly through the air. The sight below you is breathtaking.

What do you see? A winding river. The ocean dotted with islands, each island rimmed in turquoise water. You see jagged snowcapped mountain peaks. A magnificent city stretching to the horizon. You float through a bank of clouds, and it is like moving through cotton balls.

Slowly you begin your descent, gliding softly back down to earth. Swooping, gliding, backflapping your wings, you reduce the speed of your descent as the earth comes rushing toward you. You flap your wings elegantly for a perfect landing, coming to rest back in your room. You feel your wings disappear. You sit up and open your eyes, still full of feelings and wonder and ecstasy. You had no idea you could fly!

Day 68: Moving into the House of Joy

On a small piece of paper, draw a picture of a house. Make it as elaborate as you like. Make it a mansion or make it a cottage. Now close your eyes and visualize yourself opening the door to this charming and inviting house. Come into the entryway and look around. Locate all the rooms to the left and to the right of you and imagine how they are furnished. Is there an upstairs? Are there people in the rooms? What kind of activity is going on? Move from room to room and decide what the different spaces are used for—a place for everyone to dine together; a place for quiet meditating; a quiet place to sleep; a place to work, make music, dance, or just hang out and be with others.

This is the House of Joy. How many people live with you here? How many faces do you recognize? How many are strangers? Introduce yourself and find out who they are and what they are about. Open your eyes. Label the picture you drew "The House of Joy." Save it, for you will be using it in a later activity.

Day 69: Nourishing the 60 percent—From Tragedy to Comedy

Develop three jokes that you rehearse and have ready to tell at an appropriate moment. The three jokes that you add to your repertoire should be appropriate for different types of people—you don't want all three to be unsuitable for the straightlaced or when children are present. On the other hand, have prepared a much wider selection of jokes for people you are close to. Not even the best joke teller just wings it and somehow gets a laugh. Jokes are usually best told with animation and expression, and even the pauses and gestures are important. You don't have to script a joke, but you might rehearse alone before you try it out on someone—a good friend, a colleague at work, or, later on, a small group at lunch or a party. If the joke you've chosen is a dud, that doesn't mean you're not funny. The best way to tell a joke is standing up. There's more energy to it and people have a tendency to be more animated that way. Even a story is better told standing up.

Telling jokes is one of the most immediate ways you can change the way people experience you, from someone sad and troubled to someone vibrant and alive. Even if they don't laugh, the fact that your focus was on their enjoyment has radically changed the perception.

Day 70: Nourishing the 60 Percent— My Success Story

Think back on all the things you have done in your life that have made you proud—all the difficult things you have accomplished in spite of many obstacles. Think of all the difficult circumstances you have overcome. Make a list of all these past successes and give specific details.

Describe these accomplishments to someone who knows you well. Then ask, "Have I forgotten anything?" The person may then respond with some successes or attributes you may have overlooked or given insufficient value.

Answer in writing the following question: What

might be preventing me from making full use of all my attributes, talents, and strengths? Based upon the response, set yourself an immediate goal of putting your strengths to use somehow within the next week.

Ask yourself a second question: How might I use my strengths to better my meaningful relationships? Based on the response, set yourself an immediate goal of one week for doing something positive to improve one of those relationships.

Day 71: Nourishing the 60 Percent— Becoming Proactive

Choose a day when you will plan your weekly calendar. Sunday night might not suit you, but whatever day you choose, be consistent. Beginning with this week, make at least one dinner date and choose one evening of entertainment—going out to a movie; staying home to play cards; or going out to play billiards, bowl, or see a sporting event. If you ask someone who turns you down, keep calling. People are busy, but you may find that next week they may be calling you to go out. Within a few weeks of filling in your own calendar of events, I guarantee you will have broken your isolative ways.

Day 72: Response-ability—Body Stretch

This is a good daytime energy booster: Lie on the floor and close your eyes. Feel your body. Without straining, stretch every part of your body from your feet to your head—toes, feet, ankles, calves, knees, thighs, hips, stomach, chest, arms, hands, fingers, neck, head—your total body. Experience how you feel. Open your eyes.

Stand up. Imagine you are a tree with a very tall trunk and roots that go deep into the soil. Raise your arms to become branches and reach them skyward as high as they will go, each finger stretched out and reaching to the limit until you can reach no further. Imagine the sun entering through the leaves that are your fingers to become nourishment that travels down your arms, down through your legs and feet, and reaching down through your roots into the earth, grounding you.

Now give all your limbs a good shake. Feel how you are full of energy from the sun. The warmth you feel is an expression of the energy source that is your spirit. As the sun warms the earth and nourishes growing things, your spirit gives you the energy to live fully. Take that good energy into your day.

Day 73: Response-ability—What Gives You Pleasure?

In your journal, list for each of the five senses— sight, smell, touch, hearing, and taste—what gives you pleasure. Get very specific for each sense, such as exactly what kind of guitar music, acoustic or hard rock, you enjoy listening to or what types of flowers smell the sweetest. When you have finished, read over the list and describe yourself as a sensuous person, someone who experiences the physical side of life with attention and appreciation for nuances and detail, not someone who simply consumes or reacts to stimuli. Explore how you came to have such favorites in each of the five senses.

Day 74: Response-ability—A Walk

The next time you go for a walk, try this sensory enhancement activity: For a few minutes focus on the sounds you hear. Identify as many as you can. Next, focus on the smells around you and identify as many as you can. For the next few minutes, touch everything you can and note the peculiarities and the temperatures of the surfaces that you touch. Sit for a moment, pick a primary color, and find as many shades of that color as you can in the scene before you. Notice the shadows of everything and how they fall. Notice the differences in light and how it changes. Notice the clouds, if there are any, and the speed and direction at which they travel.

Close your eyes and let your sensations mingle together to create one heightened experience, in Proust's words, "an invasion of exquisite pleasures."

VII

Relationships: Loved for Who You Are

Who I Am

The first time I told someone that all I ever wanted was to be loved for who I am, I choked on the words. It is an especially poignant statement coming from a chronic doer. I really believed that I had to do something to have an identity in order to be loved and accepted by others. I really believed I was in a relationship because of what I could do, not because of who I was.

Even today, sometimes when I tell people all I ever want is to be loved for who I am, tears come to my eyes. It has the same effect on others. Each time this happens, I think, "What on earth is going on here? Deep down inside, is this really what we all want?" I believe it is, and that what is loved is our spirit, for it is who we really are. That spirit becomes our identity. You don't discover it; it was always there. Since day one of this process, you have been tearing down the walls trying to get to it, removing the masks, uncovering the secrets, and out of willingness and desire to become reconnected one day (perhaps it has already happened) your spirit will emerge in all its childlike energy, simplicity, freedom, and love for you.

People who allow their spirits to emerge are no longer hiding anything, and they become translucent. The more open they become, the more others are able to experience them, to "take them in." Becoming translucent is not the same as being transparent. Some people are open to a point that it is unbearable. We feel that they have no respect for their own privacy.

There are things that are important to keep to ourselves—not the bad things, but the good things we do. We develop strength of character and nourish our spirit when we privately do good things. I believe that keeping this part of ourselves private also keeps us interesting, even mysterious. Remember the Lone Ranger? He would do his good deed and then ride with Tonto off into the sunset, never revealing his true identity. That made people curious. They always went around asking, "Who was that masked man?" Be the Lone Ranger, and people will want to know who you really are, too.

I'm a Perfect Size 18

I once read an interview with Oprah Winfrey in which she said, "I keep trying to tell myself, you are home now, you are safe. Intellectually I know it, but not my spirit, soul, heart. Then weight will no longer be an issue.'' She is right.

Years ago I thought my body was the solution to all my problems, but body size is not the answer.

A lot of times when I tell people that I'm a perfect size 18, I get some funny looks. I have no shame in making that statement, and I don't have to apologize for who I am. I know I'm overweight in some people's eyes and that they may think I'm rationalizing or in denial. Yet, every time I really think about it, I have to conclude that I'm perfectly comfortable the way I am. I know that if I tried to become a size 16 or a size 14 that I could accomplish that, but I would be doing it for someone else and not for me, and I have a hard time rationalizing how being either size would have an impact on my life. It's not going to change my relationships, and it's not going to give me something I don't already have.

It's a matter of perception. Whenever I go to a museum and see all the voluptuous women depicted by painters through the ages, I have to laugh. If I had been born into any other century, I would be a really hot number! Today I define who I am by my own rules and standards, and from my own perception, I am a perfect size 18. That's not to say that I don't think people should be thin if they want to be, and I definitely think people should change their size if they believe their weight is affecting their health or decreasing their ability to express themselves. If you feel that way and if you are sure you want to lose weight, then by all means go for it. However, do it for yourself, not for anyone else.

Although I tell people about being a perfect size 18 because it communicates my point, it still bothers me. I'm not a size anything. I'm just me, Janet, loving, giving, caring. As Popeye the Sailorman says, "I yam who I yam."

Weight, the Last Mask Off

For many of us, extra weight was the first mask we wore to protect ourselves. Maybe it's only appropriate that weight is also the last mask off. Over sixteen years of recovery, I have noticed time and again that when people give up all their other addictions, a craving for food comes roaring forth. You might say this addiction is the last resort of many in trying to fill the emptiness left by their disconnected spirits.

Until your spirit is fully restored, weight loss will only make you feel too vulnerable, especially if you have sexual issues. I have known many people who have lost a lot of weight and felt so uncomfortable with their newly uncovered selves that they put the weight right back on. Instead of dieting, the focus should be on that emptiness you are trying to fill by eating. Instead of stepping on and off scales and measuring out food, you can be nourishing the 60 percent. Then in time, the 10 percent that is the body will take care of itself. The more you value yourself, the less you will value food until one day it will be restored to its proper place. Without your conscious effort, you will use it to nourish your body, not your spirit. Then you will never have to weigh, measure, or calculate your food again.

Intimacy, Spirit to Spirit

Whenever I ask a group of people, "How many here have enough intimacy in their lives?" invariably they all laugh. The truth is, most people have never experienced intimacy because they can't. It is impossible to connect with others until you've connected with yourself. Without your spirit, you present a stranger to a love partner, and he or she has to guess who you really are; what your needs really are; and what you are really thinking, feeling, and desiring behind your mask.

For survivors of childhood sexual abuse, the ability to experience real intimacy becomes distorted. When I was disconnected, sex was not about getting close. Quite the opposite, it was about power. I could only feel intensely about a man if I felt he was powerful, for my secret need was for protection.

Sex didn't have much to do with my body; in fact, I was hardly there. Even when I was physically close to someone, emotionally I kept him at a distance. Long ago I had learned to disassociate from anything sexual. As an adult I remained frozen. I just couldn't *feel* sexual the way most people did.

When you become reconnected, it is your spirit that experiences your sexual feelings, and the sexual act becomes an interchange of energy—spirit to spirit. In turn, energy expands our spirit, allowing us to experience a wonderful warm feeling that penetrates to our core being.

Of course, such a dramatic change in the way sexuality is experienced does not happen overnight. In the early months of my recovery, when I was overwhelmed by many things I was learning about myself, I decided to keep sex out of my relationships for a while. I learned something of value during that time. Instead of wondering whether men wanted to be with me or if they just wanted to have sex, I was able to really get to know them the way I got to know my women friends. Another astonishing discovery: Men were individuals, not an entity of badness and danger. In fact, some had really sweet personalities and were capable of many different responses. I was fascinated by how different men could be. I realized I had been doing them an injustice by reacting to them as a species that only wanted one thing from me rather than responding to them as individuals with whom I could have healthy relationships that were balanced by give and take.

In recovery, I completely reversed my approach to sex. Before, operating from a level of confusion and low self-esteem, having sex began the relationship and then I would figure where to go from there. Now it is only natural that time is spent getting to know one another before I have sex with a man. If we finally do have sex, it isn't body to body contact, it is an energy exchange between spirits. For the first time I can be truly present while having sex, for my fears have vanished like shadows in the radiance of my spirit, and I can let someone else feel that warmth.

Over the years, my priorities have changed so much that I now value intimacy, friendship, and nurturing in my relationships more than I value sex. I really believe that my cup runneth over. I have such beautiful people in my life. I am a sexual being, I feel my sensuality, and I know that I have an energy that is attractive to other people, just as I'm attracted to them.

True intimacy on any level, sexual or nonsexual, is a wonderful, powerful, and exciting energy exchange, a mutual letting in of another's spirit. Once you experience this exchange, you will understand why you have felt so lonely for so long—*a great deal has been missing!*

ACTIVITIES
Days 75-90

Day 75: The 30 Percent—Make Your Point in Thirty Seconds

Now that you have experienced your 60 percent, you are equipped to work on that part of your being that gives so much trouble in early recovery, the 30 percent of yourself that is cognitive: What you think has to play catch-up with what you "know." Although our 60 percent may be responding in ways that feel new and unique, we often find the 30 percent of ourselves responding in the same old way, as if the words just lined up one behind the other in our brain and jumped out of our mouths before we had time to stop them. Fortunately, we can train our cognitive selves with just a little practice.

I highly recommend the book *How to Get Your Point Across in Thirty Seconds or Less* by Milo O. Frank (New York: Pocket Books, 1987). It's great for people who are so insecure that they have a tendency to tell every detail of something that happens. People don't need all the details. In the movie *The Player,* screenwriters have to present their ideas for a new film to a jaded and harried studio executive in twenty-five words or less. Having to do this on the spot throws them into a tailspin. However, if those twenty-five words are hammered out in advance, they can be a great thought clarifier. Brevity empowers your message and makes the task of developing the idea much easier because it eliminates the extraneous.

When you have an idea for something that intrigues you, or if you are working on something you're really involved in, try describing it in twenty-five words or less or in thirty seconds. Or if you are having trouble getting through to someone important in your life—a spouse, boss, parent, or child—script and then rehearse making your point within the above restrictions and you will find a way to present it that both defines yourself and can be taken in by the other party.

Day 76: The 30 Percent—"What Part of No Don't You Understand?"

People who have been abused have a very hard time with boundaries, whereas some people are so defensive no one can get close to them. Others, so afraid that someone won't like them, give in too easily. It helps to have in your mind some catchy phrases that you can say out loud and tell yourself, depending on the situation, when someone refuses to acknowledge what you are saying, is convinced they have to change your mind, or threatens your boundaries in any way. Try: "What part of *no* don't you understand?" Or "No is a complete sentence."

Rehearse your responses in front of a mirror. People often get a lot of enjoyment out of this exercise.

Another boundary situation that makes a lot of peo-

ple uncomfortable is being probed to tell more than
they want to disclose. One of the great comforts of
recovery is learning you don't have to tell all, or anything, if you wish to respect your privacy or the privacy of others. Practice the following responses to a
probing question: "I just don't know what to say."
"I'm wondering why you're asking me that."

Or you may try the tactic of diversion. Simply ig-
nore the question and change the subject: "Who do
you think is going to win the election?" "How is the
addition on your house coming along?"

You may find that firming up your boundaries
makes some people all the more determined to cross
them, particularly when you allowed them that privilege before. If they persist, rehearse these responses
calmly, politely, and with dignity: "I couldn't possibly comment on that." "I really don't want to have
this conversation."

The next time you find yourself in an uncomfortable boundary situation, remember these scripted responses. You may not even use them but
acknowledging your discomfort has in itself fortified
those boundaries, and in that newfound serenity, the
words you need may not require any searching at all.

Day 77: The 10 Percent

Sometimes your body expresses itself more effec-
tively than words. Unlike verbal communication, the
body gives a true indication of feelings while words
can lie about and conceal those true feelings. To get
an idea of how expressive your body can be in communicating with others, stand in front of a mirror and

repeat the scripted responses from yesterday's activity. Then communicate each response without words. When you are restricted verbally, you give your body a chance to express what you mean. I think you will be amazed how much it communicates without your needing to say anything at all.

Day 78: The 40 (10 + 30) Percent—"You've Got It? Good!"

Communicating with Intention

Communications often fail because participants do not fully acknowledge and communicate their intentions clearly through words as well as body language, employing both the 10 and 30 percents. As a result, people often don't get what they want or need. Script your intentions in preparation for an encounter with someone with whom you are having difficulty communicating:

Stand up and look in a mirror. Concentrate on standing firmly and maintaining eye contact with yourself, because during the encounter you will make eye contact with the other person. When you speak the words, do something with your body that demonstrates your feelings.

Address the person by name. Tell him or her, "I need _____." For example, "I need some time alone for myself today." You might cross your arms or turn your back. Try expressing your needs again, using different words and body language. The goal of this interchange is to hear from the other person, "I understand." Then you know there has been a real connection. Sometimes you may say, "Do you understand?" and hear "Yes, but . . ." in reply. Try another way of expressing your need until the person tells you, "I've got it."

Day 79: The People Pleasers Boycott

People pleasers have a hard time withdrawing from their need to have others like them. They are often so shame based that their verbal reactions are knee-jerk. If someone bumps into them they will say, "I'm sorry." I have even seen people pleasers apologize to lampposts, dogs, and trees! These apologies are harmful because they give us away. In effect, we announce to the world that we believe we are guilty of something and are willing to assume blame indiscriminately. That can be a dangerous message to put out about ourselves. For the next forty-eight hours, declare a ban on saying "I'm sorry."

When the forty-eight hours are up, write your reactions in your journal. Describe how you felt at the moment when you refrained from speaking the forbidden phrase. Panic? Terror? Fear? Discomfort? Those feelings belong to your former self with its core of shame, not you.

Were there times when the phrase "I'm sorry" escaped from your mouth in spite of your best intentions? How did those lapses makes you feel? Angry? Scared? Like a robot? Your automatic "I'm sorry" is just a habit you can unlearn. The panic button that could previously summon those words unbidden can be nicely unwired.

Extend your forty-eight-hour moratorium for as long as you need to until you no longer feel that involuntary urge to apologize or can recognize it in time to silence it. Eventually, when you really do want to say "I'm sorry," the words will hold more meaning; they will emanate not cheaply from a shame-based core, but with value from your spirit, which wants you to transcend the hurtful plane.

Day 80: Asking Questions

This exercise is for control freaks. If you have come far enough on your journey that you can say, "That's me!" then here is a simple tool you can employ every time you are in a conversation with someone. If you're not a control freak, you might try this scripted activity anyway. The goal is to make any exchange a fifty–fifty proposition, spirit to spirit:

Think of five people you talk to often. In your journal, write down a question that would be appropriate to ask each of the five people. Choose something you know is their passion, their heart's desire, or at least their interest. Here are some examples: "How is the quilt coming along?" "How's the new baby?" "Have you finished the extension on the house?"

Now write down a second question for each of the five people, this time asking their advice. Keep these questions in mind.

The next time you talk, either in person or on the phone, use the following scenario:

After the appropriate greetings, ask your first question. As the person responds, keep conscious track of the time. Make a mental note of it. When the person winds down, he or she may go on to another subject. Let it happen. It is at this point that the false person you were, the control freak, goes into a tailspin. You've *got* to be in control of that conversation! Take some deep breaths and relax. Let your spirit be in charge.

At a certain point, the person will ask you about yourself. Then allow yourself whatever amount of time the other person took, less if you can. Then ask your second question. Everyone feels good about being asked for advice: what shade to paint the kitchen, what kind of car or rug to buy, what doctor they should see. Unlike doing a favor, giving advice is effortless and most people feel good about being asked for their opinion.

If you feel a lot of resistance to this assignment, know that it's not about letting go of the control but letting in your spirit. Give it half a chance and it will take over. As the conversation is taking place, note how you are feeling. Does the other person seem animated, cheerful, in need of being heard out? Are you really listening? Or are you just pretending to listen, waiting for a break in the conversation to jump in and take over as you used to? As you listen, try to hear what the person needs.

Repeat this mental exercise until the rule of fifty–fifty becomes comfortable. I think you will be gratified by the new way others respond to you and the richer quality of your relationships.

Day 81: Behind the Mask

You already have the materials necessary for making a mask from Day Sixty. There should be enough gauze to make another. Follow the same steps for making this mask, but don't decorate it. Instead, paint it black or white. It is a mask without facial features, only holes for you to see through.

After your second mask is complete, put it next to your spirit mask and perform the following activity.

Put on your new mask and look in the mirror. Make the following statement: "This is the mask I show the world when I am afraid."

Demonstrate with your body how you protect yourself when you are fearful. Using words, describe the situations in which fear comes up for you.

Now take your spirit mask and make the following statement: "This is what my spirit does when I am afraid."

Demonstrate once more by word and gesture how your spirit helps, comforts, and encourages you.

Take this mask that you hide behind when you are fearful, this mask that keeps people from getting close to you and that keeps you from being able to get close to others, and throw it in the garbage.

Write in your journal how you felt about doing this activity. What situations still make you fearful? What would it take to let go of that fear? What benefits can you reap from dropping the mask you hide behind when you are fearful?

Day 82: Patterns

Listed below are a few of the most common power plays that sabotage relationships. Check each statement you identify with in your relationships. Make two check marks where it is true in more than one relationship:

In my relationship(s), I have experienced either myself or my partner as

_____ 1. Giving advice, with difficulty taking it.

_____ 2. Having difficulty in reaching out and asking for support and love.

_____ 3. Giving orders and demanding and expecting too much from the other.

_____ 4. Trying to "get even" or to diminish the self- esteem or power of the other.

_____ 5. Tending to be judgmental, using put-downs that sabotage the other's success, fault-finding, persecuting, punishing.

_____ 6. "Holding out" on the other, not giving what the other wants or needs.

_____ 7. Making, then breaking promises.

_____ 8. Smothering or overnurturing the other.

_____ 9. Patronizing, condescending treatment of the other that sets one partner up as superior and the other as inferior; intimidation.

_____10. Making decisions for the other and discounting the other's ability to problem-solve.

_____11. Having difficulty admitting mistakes or saying "I'm sorry."

_____12. Giving indirect, evasive answers to questions.

_____13. Manipulating to put the other in no-win situations.

_____14. Attempting to change the other (but unwilling to change the self).

If you answered yes to more than half these questions, you might find the following activity helpful.

Day 83: Patterns—What I Remember

Read through the section of your notebook "What I Remember" and see if you can find any patterns in the memories you have been writing down—in your motivations or expectations. Read through the journal you have been keeping, looking for similar themes, scenarios that keep repeating, relationships that begin and end in the same way, or similarities in the characteristics of the people you choose to have in your life.

I was in recovery for many years before I saw the pattern in my life of choosing to love men who I thought would protect me. My true feelings were that deeply hidden. Once I saw the pattern, however, I was shocked at how obvious the clues were. Each husband fitted perfectly in the role of protector, a role I so desperately needed to fill. I was saddened by all the unhappiness my unconscious motivations had caused myself and others. Patterns are so difficult to recognize because we'd rather not know how much we do for unconscious reasons. However, we must know in order to make the behavior conscious so we can stop doing damage to ourselves and others.

Another example of a pattern is common among women who were victims of incest by their fathers. It is the love triangle, with an unavailable man standing in for the father, and the wife, fiancée, or current girlfriend representing the mother from whom the affair must be kept a secret. Repeaters of this pattern often say they feel real excitement only in playing the role of the "other woman" in circumstances that are forbidden, re-creating their childhood dilemma over and over, trying to resolve it but unable to see the pattern, let alone break out of it.

Loss of opportunity, or situations in which people

with low self-esteem repeatedly "snatch defeat from the jaws of victory," is another common example of a pattern. At a crucial moment, the person misses a plane, gets ill, or has an accident or an emotional flare-up that results in the loss of opportunity. This pattern of self-sabotage is common because so many people believe in their core being that they don't deserve good things.

If you don't see a pattern right away, keep trying. Pay attention to those feelings of "Uh-oh, here I go again." Sooner or later, if there is a hidden pattern in your life and you are honest with yourself, you will find it.

Day 84: Old Friends

In your journal, make a list of the people you are close to. For each person, note down the length of time you have been close. Describe the frequency of contact and whether there have been gaps in that contact during the time you have known them. Describe your oldest friend. What is it about this person that makes you close? How do you value your friends, and what contributions have they made to your life? What does the quality of your relationships say about you?

Day 85: Happiness Index

Take out the roll of paper on which you illustrated your time line on Day Twenty and spread it on a table or floor. You are now going to give it a happiness index. With the top of the paper representing the most happy and the bottom of the paper representing the least happy, graph your current perception of your state of mind from birth to present. If you were particularly happy at a certain point, make a dot relatively close to the top of the page; a sadder period would be indicated by a dot near the bottom. Now connect all the dots.

When you are through graphing your happiness index, describe it in your journal. Did the line you drew have a lot of peaks and valleys, or was it pretty much in the middle? What was your highest peak? Your lowest low? Were there more highs than lows, or the other way around? Judging by the line, would you say your life so far has been mostly happy? Mostly unhappy? Or has it been a numb straight line down the middle of the paper? Write about the happiest time. What qualities did it have? Describe your environment of that time—the house, tree, yard, community. What is missing today? How could you get that quality into your life today?

Hang your chart on the wall for a while. It takes time to absorb the bigger picture. With the chart on the wall, some say they feel like generals in a war room plotting the defense of a nation. I think they're doing something more important: They are protecting their spirit. Study your chart and note how happy your life has been thus far. Consider where you are now and know that you have the power to direct your life on the path toward happiness. Use your chart to learn from your past and chart how you'd like your future to be.

Or you may want to keep your chart on the wall for a while for a completely different reason. For you it may be a trophy, a victory of self-determination over difficult obstacles, and the present moment, your just reward.

One day when you get tired of looking at your time line and want the wall space for other things, roll it up and put it away. Over the years this time line will grow in meaning for you, and you will want to keep it to chart the future.

Day 86: The Community of Joy

On Day Sixty-eight you drew a small picture of your House of Joy. Take this picture and on a large sheet of paper draw a community around it until you have a small village—in the country or a big city—whatever you decide. Describe in your journal how, as part of a Community of Joy, you take from that community and how you give back.

Day 87: The Sacred Tree

The Tree of Life is one of the most ancient of human symbols, signifying growth and communion with nature. Find a tree that to you symbolizes this growth and this connection. Maybe it is in your front yard, down the street, or in a city park. Wherever it is, declare that tree sacred to you. Sit under that tree and contemplate how you and it are similar—in growth, endurance, beauty, stillness—whatever the tree imparts to you that resonates in your spirit. Put your arms around the tree and allow yourself to let in the message that you are a good person. If it is hard for you to take that message in, hug the tree a little: endurance, dignity, and strength.

Day 88: Who Am I Now?

In your journal describe the changes that have taken place since you began your journey eighty-seven days ago. What secrets have you discovered? What questions have been answered? How has the change affected your relationships, your work, your peace of mind? What issues remain unresolved? Ask your spirit for guidance in taking action.

Day 89: Epitaph

I recently saw a *New Yorker* cartoon that really made me laugh. It was a picture of a tombstone with the epitaph "Never sick a day in his life and now this." Death is a reality, but what's more important is what you did with your life. Saying what that life was all about with the brevity and wit of an epitaph is a way to describe your essence—that intangible thing about you that makes you so exciting. However, epitaphs aren't easy. Like poetry, you don't just sit down and come up with several words that best describe who you are and what your life is about.

The visionary architect Buckminster Fuller's epitaph is "Call Me Trimtab," a nautical expression for maneuvering a craft through the waves with minimum resistance. It's a wonderfully accurate metaphor for the inventor of the geodesic dome, but I bet he didn't come up with it overnight.

How would you like your epitaph to read? Think about it.

Day 90: Reconnecting—A Guided Imagery

The following exercise is preceded by deep breathing or the progressive relaxation exercise. Allow plenty of time. Lie comfortably and close your eyes:

Experience yourself walking in a forest. Notice the sights and sounds around you. What do you smell? What do you see? What do you hear? What do you feel? You are surrounded by beauty and serenity. You are struggling somehow to connect with your peaceful surroundings, yet something seems to be preventing you from doing this. Something is preventing you from being able to enjoy the here and now.

You continue to walk in this beautiful peaceful forest and come to a gate attached to a long high wall. You approach the gate and open it slowly. As you walk through the gate, you look up to see a huge, ugly, smelly junk pile. Notice what you are feeling as you experience this odious, rotting stack of garbage.

Keeping your eyes closed, sit up, then stand up. Place your internal junk on the junk pile. You may throw it in or kick it in. Keeping your eyes closed, take the time now to let go of *all* your junk, every bit of it. Feel around in the corners and under and behind things, but do whatever it takes to clean out all your junk so you can leave it on this big stinking pile and get away from it because the smell is really getting to you.

Lie down again. Walk back to the gate, walk

through it, and go back along the path through the forest. Notice a big sign that says Danger: Junk Pile Decomposition Site. Know that the big pile of smelly junk is being transformed by an environmental cleanup crew into harmless compost out beyond the forest where it can't pollute the air or soil and make people ill.

Notice how you feel as you walk through the forest this time. Is there any difference? The forest leads to an open meadow where there is grass, clover, flowers, sunshine, rabbits, deer, soothing breezes, sounds of birds, fragrances, a rippling brook. Experience whatever joy and serenity you would like in this meadow. Allow yourself to frolic and play freely and spontaneously.

Now it's time to leave. Know you can come back to this meadow anytime you wish.

In your journal, write down anything you may not have been able to throw on the junk pile. What do you think it would take to rid yourself of this piece of toxic waste?

Know you can do this visualization anytime you are ready to dispose of it. Every time you visit this meadow, you will feel lighter and more filled with your spirit.

Afterthoughts

THE VALLEY OF LOVE AND DELIGHT

It's a gift to be simple
It's a gift to be free
It's a gift to be
Where we ought to be
And when we find ourselves
In the place just right
It will be in the valley
of Love and Delight.

The above lines from Aaron Copland's adaptation
of the Shaker hymn "Simple Gifts" contain the vision
I have for you, but this wonderful place is not a destination—it is who you really are. It is the great and
unexpected gift of recovery. At "Your Life Matters,"
we have received incredible feedback from patients
and readers of my first book, recounting specific
things that have happened to change their lives for
the better. Because they now value themselves, other
people value them. They aspire to things they had
never dreamed of. They have started their own busi-
nesses, written their own books, feel empowered in
their jobs, don't feel stuck in fear. They don't have

the craziness of looking for magic or of looking to food as a solution. Many describe how not just their own lives, but the lives of everyone around them, have changed for the better.

It is my deepest hope that this book will also change your life for the better and that it has already helped you experience who you are and the *power* of who you are. This may be the end of the book, but it's the beginning of a wonderful journey. If you allow yourself to continue on this journey, it will take you beyond your wildest dreams and fill your life with love and delight.

Acknowledgments

We can do no great things,
only little things with great love.

—Mother Teresa

No one can write a book alone. This book was made possible by the love of God and Saint Theresa, "the little flower." It grew out of the combined support of precious friends who refused to give up on me year after year. Their devotion and relentless energy go far beyond mere gratitude, but I will try.

First, Catherine Revland is holding a reservation for a front-row seat in heaven, I'm sure of it. She's an angel. Without Catherine's wisdom, the preceding pages would still be dancing inside my head. She and God made it all make sense.

I am blessed to have the gentle, warm love and intelligence of my mother reflected in these pages and in my life. The strength, love, and bursting good humor of my children, Gene, Jimmy, and Roe, kept me going when I couldn't find anything funny. They have always been there for me and have made my life wonderfully exciting.

How very fortunate I am to have Budd Holden and

Andre Poit as real friends who inspire me to remain "God's kid" always. I see God's love reflected in them every day with love, life, and truth.

Love is experienced in many ways, and because "Your Life Matters" is really God's company, He put wonderful angels in my life and on my staff: Kitty Duffy's love and trust, Marty Van Herik's warm friendship, Deneice Howard's compassion, Fred Earle's loving spirit, Beatrice Cohen's humor, Jann Sellers' warmth, Bob Crane's spontaneity, Paige Hargrove's shining light, Kim Comeau's abundant energy, Jack Ayala's loving spark, Larry Dean's loyalty, Jerry Smith's dedication, Peggy Favata's kindness, Roland Mora's kindred spirit, and Tom Bell's love. Let me not forget past husbands who have made my life interesting and fun.

I will be forever grateful to my editor, Denise Silvestro, who captured this book in her own delicate and sensitive way. My deep appreciation always to my agent, Frank Weimann.

Special love to all present and past staff of "Your Life Matters," who have dedicated themselves to make a difference in the lives of others. You are all God's kids and you make the difference. I also thank Mother Teresa, Dr. Robert Schuller, Oprah, and Joan Rivers, who have impacted my life indirectly but in a remarkable way.

I dedicate this book to you. It's your book now! My dream is that it will empower you to be all that you can be.

For information about Janet Greeson's
"Your Life Matters"
Please call 1-800-515-1995